HIGH INCOME CAN BE A MIXED BLESSING. DON'T LOSE IT . . . LEARN TO ACCUMULATE IT. THIS PROFESSIONAL GUIDE TO FINANCIAL SUCCESS PROVIDES:

- Self-diagnostic reviews to help you evaluate your overall financial profile
- Tools to organize your personal records
- Debt management and spending control
- Tips on insurance coverage and tax breaks especially for doctors, dentists, and health-care professionals
- The best investment portfolio for you
- Retirement objectives and plans
- Work sheets and action plans
- Ten simple things to do to help you achieve financial peace of mind in the 1990s
  . . . AND MORE

COMPLETE, COMPREHENSIVE, AND PERSONALIZED

POND'S
PERSONALIZED FINANCIAL PLANNING GUIDE FOR
DOCTORS, DENTISTS, AND HEALTH-CARE PROFESSIONALS

Look for these other Pond's Personalized Financial Planning Guides
by Jonathan D. Pond

■

POND'S PERSONALIZED FINANCIAL PLANNING GUIDE FOR
SALESPEOPLE

■

POND'S PERSONALIZED FINANCIAL PLANNING GUIDE FOR SELF-
EMPLOYED PROFESSIONALS AND SMALL BUSINESS OWNERS

■

POND'S PERSONALIZED FINANCIAL PLANNING GUIDE FOR
TEACHERS AND EMPLOYEES OF EDUCATIONAL INSTITUTIONS

POND'S PERSONALIZED FINANCIAL PLANNING GUIDE FOR DOCTORS, DENTISTS, AND HEALTH-CARE PROFESSIONALS

JONATHAN D. POND

A DELL TRADE PAPERBACK

A DELL TRADE PAPERBACK

Published by
Dell Publishing
a division of
Bantam Doubleday Dell Publishing Group, Inc.
666 Fifth Avenue
New York, New York 10103

The trademark Dell® is registered in the U.S. Patent and Trademark Office.

ISBN: 0-440-50394-9

Design: Stanley S. Drate/Folio Graphics Co., Inc.

Printed in the United States of America

Published simultaneously in Canada

September 1991

10 9 8 7 6 5 4 3 2 1

RRC

To Elizabeth

ACKNOWLEDGMENTS

Numerous people have participated in the preparation of this book, although they may not realize how helpful they have been. Over the past decade I have spoken and worked with many physicians, dentists, and health-care professionals. While each may have thought that his or her individual financial circumstances were unique, there is a great deal of commonality of financial needs among members of the health-care profession. This book focuses on those shared needs and concerns.

Viveca Gardiner was instrumental in assisting with the research and preparation of this book, and her many contributions are gratefully acknowledged.

I also sincerely appreciate the wonderful and insightful guidance of my two editors at Dell, Jody Rein and Jeanne Cavelos.

My family was very understanding of my long absences. Perhaps special recognition should be given to my new daughter, Laura, who arrived on the scene in the midst of my writing. Without her "help" this book would have been published several months earlier.

CONTENTS

INTRODUCTION

People spend more time thinking about personal money matters than they do thinking about any other single subject, according to a recent survey. I know from my work that people do worry a lot about their personal finances, but even I thought money matters would rank second as far as what adults like to think about. Personal financial planning is an important subject for everyone. After all, we work hard for our money, and we want to retire comfortably. Yet turning that money into financial security is no easy task, and it's made even harder by the perception of the complexity of personal finance and by our daily bombardment with often conflicting, often biased financial advice. In the course of counseling members of various occupations on financial planning matters, it occurred to me that working in a particular occupation presents a variety of unique financial planning opportunities and problems. For example, in my work counseling medical professionals, I have found that although many of them earn substantial incomes, they tend to adjust their life-styles, fully expecting that their incomes will continue to rise forever. However, prospects aren't so rosy for the health-care system in this country, and many will regret not having begun to spend less and save more.

This book, directed solely to the money concerns of health-care professionals, will help you address your own personal circumstances so that it will be easier for you to take action to achieve financial security. Whether you are a doctor, dentist, or other health-care professional,* it will help you to do a better job

---

*Health-care professionals also include, but are not limited to, registered nurses and licensed practical nurses, therapists, health technologists and technicians, doctors' and dental assistants, and other people who are employed by health-care institutions.

with your money. While health-care professionals aren't much different from members of other occupations—insofar as everyone wants to achieve financial security—medical professionals do share some unique characteristics that can and should influence the course of your personal financial planning. For example:

■ Many enjoy higher-than-average income, which can be a mixed blessing. On one hand, higher incomes provide the opportunity to invest more money in a variety of attractive investment products and retirement plans. On the other hand, a high income that is accompanied by high spending can be dangerous to your financial health.

■ Many health-care professionals are self-employed, and therefore can avail themselves of a number of advantageous retirement plans and other tax-beneficial transactions.

■ Many health-care professionals are employed by nonprofit organizations, which have somewhat different, yet very attractive retirement plans.

■ Because of their professional endeavors and prominence in the community, many health-care professionals have unique insurance needs.

■ The health-care system in this country is likely to experience some major changes in the future, most of which do not bode well for people who work in the profession. These prospects should influence the financial planning process of medical professionals.

Many medical professionals put off their financial planning or think their finances are under control, when, in fact, they may not be. This book contains a variety of work sheets and self-diagnostic reviews that can help you understand where you stand. Even if you find that you are in relatively good financial health, you will find numerous suggestions in these pages that will help you do a better job.

While money is the focal point, successful personal financial planning encompasses a variety of areas, including:

■ Setting financial objectives and planning to meet them
■ Organizing your personal records
■ Managing your debt effectively and bringing your spending under control
■ Saving and investing regularly

- Accumulating an investment portfolio that meets your needs
- Minimizing income taxes
- Planning to achieve a comfortable retirement
- Preparing and maintaining appropriate estate planning documents.

All of these topics and more will be covered in this book. The advantage of reading a book written just for medical professionals is that you won't have to wade through a lot of material that doesn't pertain to your unique circumstances. This is not a get-rick-quick book; however, it is a get-rich-*sensibly* book. You will find a lot of common sense on these pages, because common sense is the key to successful personal financial planning. Even if you rely on financial advisors to handle much of your planning, you will still benefit by reading this book, because no matter how much you rely on others to assist you, you need to take control of your financial future.

Don't be surprised if you find the financial planning process to be rather daunting. There is a lot to be done, even if your finances are in pretty good shape. The work sheets and action plans will help you identify areas that need attention. You won't be able to do everything, and those matters that need attention cannot be addressed all at once. But begin to do one or a few things, and you will find that you *can* improve your personal financial status, and that it isn't such a burden after all. In fact, it should be fun to watch your investments grow, to know that your debt and spending are under control, to know that you are adequately insured, and to realize that you will be able to enjoy a long and financially fruitful retirement.

Financial peace of mind, like good health, requires at least some effort. You need to follow some basic rules. You need to avoid perilous activities. You need to identify warning signals and take appropriate action. If you don't follow the rules, the quality of your later life will suffer, and while you need to rely on professional assistance from time to time, only you know how you want to structure your financial life. Your basic goals and desires are the center of your personal financial life. This book will help you to translate these goals into financial terms and to achieve them, buying you a lifetime of good wealth.

I

GETTING ORGANIZED

1

Isn't It Time to Assess Your Personal Financial Health?

Why do doctors, dentists, and other health-care professionals need their own money book? Many people would probably guess, erroneously, that since medical professionals make so much money, they need to learn about fancy investment techniques and elaborate tax-avoidance strategies that don't apply to common people. That's not what this book is about. If you have fallen for fancy investment strategies, and if you have been stuck with grandiose tax shelters, this book will help alleviate your suffering. If, on the other hand, you are one of the majority in your profession who doesn't earn an income sufficient to support a family of fifty comfortably, this book will help guide you through the process of achieving financial peace of mind by recognizing that people in the medical profession do have some unique problems—and opportunities.

This book is written especially for you. It won't burden you with matters that pertain to people in other occupations or whose general financial circumstances are very different from yours. In fact, each chapter highlights those areas that are unique to medical professionals, and more importantly, each chapter will tell you how to take advantage of the financial problems that are relevant to members of your profession.

THE ANATOMY OF PERSONAL FINANCIAL PLANNING

Successful personal financial planning requires attention to three distinct yet interrelated areas: getting organized, ac-

3

cumulating wealth, and planning for later life. Within each area, there are several important matters that you should be concerned about. These will be discussed in the chapters that follow.

I. Getting Organized
- Setting financial objectives, planning to meet them, and revising them when your circumstances change
- Determining where you stand financially
- Putting your personal records in order
- Taking control of your financial future
- Finding competent financial advisers
- Acquiring and maintaining comprehensive and cost-effective insurance coverage
- Planning to meet major expenses
- Managing your debt effectively
- Bringing your spending under control

II. Accumulating Wealth
- Saving and investing regularly
- Setting realistic investment objectives
- Learning to take advantage of the numerous investment alternatives available
- Accumulating an investment portfolio that meets your needs
- Managing your investment portfolio
- Minimizing current income taxes
- Planning to reduce future income taxes

III. Planning for Later Life
- Starting to plan early for a comfortable retirement
- Projecting retirement income and expenses
- Taking advantage of tax-advantaged retirement plans
- Coordinating your retirement income needs with your personal and pension plan investments
- Making sure your estate planning documents are valid and up-to-date
- Determining if more elaborate estate planning techniques will benefit you and your heirs
- Dealing with the problems of old age—both yours and your parents'

You may think that the seemingly vast number of items listed above would require that you work full time just on your personal finances. But as you will see in this chapter and the chapters that follow, personal financial planning really isn't that complicated (although a lot of financial institutions and financial planners would like you to believe otherwise). All it takes is some discipline, a little time, and the willingness either to be your own financial planner or to make sure your financial planning adviser(s) is acting in your best interests. If successful financial planning can be boiled down to two words, they are *common sense*. If you think back on the dumb things you have done with your money in the past, and medical professionals are most definitely not immune from doing dumb things with their money on occasion, you will find that the debacles were caused by lapses of common sense. I hope you find a lot of common sense in these pages. If you're looking for no-risk ways to get rich quickly, read no further. If you're looking for ways to get rich sensibly or to be able to achieve lifetime financial security by the time you retire, you'll benefit from the advice that follows.

DECIDING WHAT YOU WANT TO ACCOMPLISH

> Two things in life that you had better not think of in financial terms: children and pets. Example: If I had a $10,000 car, I wouldn't spend ten times that amount, or $100,000, on repairs. But I just spent $250 for an eye operation on my $25 dog.

SETTING GOALS

One thing you should be doing if you haven't already is to establish some financial planning goals. What do you want to accomplish in your financial life? Permit me to tell you what your primary financial planning goal is: financial security. Financial security means that you can live the rest of your life without having to work. Most people don't achieve financial security until they retire, and there is nothing wrong with this. What is unfortunate, however, is the number of people who never achieve financial security—not by age sixty-five, not by age seventy-five, never. Don't think that just because you work in an occupation that offers both job security, and for many, high pay, that you will automatically achieve financial security. Achieving financial security requires a lot of planning and some sacrifice, because the only way you're going to be successful in reaching the universal goal of financial security (short of marrying very well or inheriting very well) is to save regularly. The only way to save regularly is to spend less than you earn, which in essence means that you have to *live beneath your means*.

Beyond the long-term goal of financial security, you probably have a variety of other financial planning objectives. Among the more common are:

- Saving more regularly
- Improving personal record keeping
- Making sure that savings are invested wisely
- Reducing debt
- Assuring complete insurance coverage
- Buying a home
- Purchasing or starting a practice
- Making a major purchase
- Reducing income taxes
- Meeting the children's college education costs
- Retiring early
- Providing support for elderly parents
- Transferring assets to children
- Making sure the estate is properly planned

You should be pretty specific about the goals you have and how you plan to go about achieving them. Be sure to write them down from time to time. To encourage you to do this, the following work sheet provides space for you to list your personal financial goals. Your most important goal has already been entered.

COPING WITH LIFE EVENTS

Over the course of your lifetime, you will experience several life events that will probably require you to reevaluate your personal financial status and plans. They will usually require you to make some adjustment in your planning, and some—divorce, for example—may require major changes. The following table lists those life events that most commonly require at least some modification of your plans.

You will note that many of the circumstances are quite common. In fact, you could lead a very typical life and experience eight to ten such events.

The nature and extent of changes required by these events vary. For some, you will need the counsel of competent professionals, but they usually cannot be expected to address all necessary changes. While it is difficult to generalize about such a

---

FINANCIAL GOALS WORK SHEET
Date: _____

1. Achieve financial security by age _____.
2. _____
3. _____
4. _____
5. _____
6. _____
7. _____

---

multiplicity of events, the following financial planning areas are often affected by the changed circumstances.

Budgeting and record keeping. Review/revise personal budgets, prepare projections, including income tax ramifications, based on changed status.

Insurance. Review beneficiary designations, adequacy of coverage, and type of coverage.

Credit. Establish or reestablish credit standing, revise loan documentation.

Family assets. Review holdings, change ownership designations, evaluate sufficiency of diversification.

Estate planning. Review/revise estate planning documents and estate planning techniques, clarify/change bequests to heirs.

MINIMIZING MARITAL MONEY SQUABBLES

When was the last time you argued with your spouse or significant other about money? If you want to have an argument, money matters are an omnipresent and very convenient catalyst. But money disputes are not necessarily indicative of deeper problems. Actually, the vast majority of couples agree on important, longer-term family financial matters. The disagreements tend to be over smaller, day-to-day financial matters. There are a couple of easy things you can do to minimize interspousal money tensions.

First, you should set aside one day every year to sit down with your spouse, review your financial status, and make some

---

TABLE 1

Life Events That Usually Require a Modification in Financial Plans

---

FAMILY
Marriage
Birth or adoption of children
Family member with special financial needs
Aging parents
Death of a spouse or other close family member
Receipt of an inheritance
Cohabitation
Separation or divorce

OCCUPATIONAL
Beginning a career
Purchasing or starting a private practice
Changing jobs or careers
Returning to school for additional training
Job subject to fluctuating income
Self-employment
Unemployment

HEALTH
Disability
Old age
Chronic illness
Terminal illness

---

plans for the next year. The date you select shouldn't be around tax-return preparation time, however. That's already stressful enough on couples. Efficient and comprehensive record keeping throughout the year will make this "day of reckoning" much easier.

Second, you should work with your spouse to develop the financial goals that were discussed earlier in this chapter. Most financial matters don't just take care of themselves. To accomplish your goals, you will have to know what they are and work toward them together.

What all this boils down to, of course, is improved communication with your spouse. Lack of communication about family finances, or for that matter, in any aspect of marriage, is a recipe for strife. But don't expect the arguments to go away entirely. Chances are you and your spouse will always have somewhat different approaches toward family money management. In fact, it you think about it, spenders tend to marry savers. While these couples may never eliminate marital money strife completely, they can, with a little communication, turn these bellicose extremes into a happier median.

Show me a married couple who has never had an argument about money, and I'll show you a couple on the way to their wedding reception.

BEING HAPPY WITH WHAT YOU'VE GOT

There is far too much preoccupation with money these days. Most people waste a lot of time thinking they would be on Easy Street if they only earned $10,000 more than they do currently. What a difference a generation makes. Our parents were certainly more content. What's so wrong with being happy with what we've got?

We all want financial security, of course. Believe it or not, some people spend all they earn during their working years thinking that they'll be able to live off Social Security when they're retired. But Social Security will support most people only about one week of each month. Assuming you'd like to provide for the other three weeks as well, you must accumulate a sizable investment portfolio by the time you retire. In order to have investments, you have to save regularly. In order to save regularly, you have to spend less than you earn.

No matter how obvious that sounds, many of us have difficulty doing it, but the best way to spend less than you earn is to be happy with what you've got. A lot of people don't like to hear this. They want a fancier car or an imported kitchen or an exotic vacation or a larger house. After all, the advertisers tell us that we have to have these things to be happy, and by golly, our neighbors have some of these things, and they sure seem happy. That's baloney, of course. The neighbors, even the ones who do make $10,000 more per year than you do, probably feel the same way about you that you feel about them. But if you can be happy with what you've got, you'll find it a lot easier to save the money to make the investments that will allow you to achieve financial security. It's as simple as that.

SETTING YOUR RECORDS STRAIGHT

Medical professionals know how important it is to maintain good records at the hospital or office. Why, then, are their personal records often in need of resuscitation? Perhaps because they are not aware of how simple an effective home record-keeping system can be. A good system is one that is comprehensive enough to be effective, yet simple enough to encourage regular use. You should think of organizing your records around three basic files: a safe-deposit box, a home active file, and an inactive file. The following Personal Record-Keeping Organizer work sheet will guide you in the process of organizing your home records.

Your *safe-deposit box* should include most of your legal and important personal papers, ownership records, and estate planning documents. Keep an updated list of the contents of the safe-deposit box in your active file. Incidentally, if you store valuables in your safe-deposit box, did you know that the bank probably doesn't insure them? You need to obtain a safe-deposit box insurance floater through the company that handles your home-owner's or renter's insurance.

Use an *active file* to monitor your current budget, organize bills, keep track of important papers, and help you in preparing the current year's tax return. Remember that if your filing system is not easy to use, you will end up postponing filing items, sometimes indefinitely. A good home active file could consist of nothing more than a cardboard box with manila file folders. You'll save time as well as money, since the chances of overlooking valuable tax deductions are smaller if your records are in order. Good personal records will also help you to avoid problems if you are ever audited by the IRS.

If you maintained your files at the hospital or office like you maintain your files at home, you'd be unemployable.

PERSONAL RECORD-KEEPING ORGANIZER

This work sheet serves two purposes. First, you can indicate next to each item where that particular item is now located. Second, you can organize your personal records by consolidating your documents into the three "files" noted below.

I. ITEMS FOR STORAGE IN SAFE-DEPOSIT BOX

PERSONAL
1. Family birth certificates _____
2. Family death certificates _____
3. Marriage certificate _____
4. Citizenship papers _____
5. Adoption papers _____
6. Veteran's papers _____
7. Social Security verification _____

OWNERSHIP
1. Bonds and certificates _____
2. Deeds _____
3. Automobile titles _____
4. Household inventories _____
5. Home-ownership records
   (e.g., blueprints, deeds, surveys,
   capital addition records, yearly records)
6. Copies of trust documents _____

OBLIGATION/CONTRACT
1. Contracts
2. Copies of insurance policies _____
3. IOUs _____
4. Retirement and pension-plan documents _____

COPIES OF ESTATE PLANNING DOCUMENTS
1. Wills _____
2. Living wills _____
3. Trusts _____
4. Letters of instruction _____
5. Guardianship arrangements _____

II. ITEMS FOR STORAGE IN HOME ACTIVE FILE

CURRENT INCOME/EXPENSE DOCUMENTS
1. Unpaid bills   _____
2. Current bank statements _____
3. Current broker's statements _____
4. Current canceled checks and money-order
   receipts _____
5. Credit card information _____

CONTRACTUAL DOCUMENTS
1. Loan statements and payment books _____
2. Appliance manuals and warranties
   (including date and place of purchase) _____
3. Insurance policies:
   - Home _____
   - Life _____
   - Automobile _____
   - Personal liability _____
   - Health and medical _____
   - Other: _____ _____
4. Receipts for expensive items not yet paid for _____

PERSONAL
1. Employment records _____
2. Health and benefits information _____
3. Family health records _____
4. Copies of wills _____
5. Copies of letters of instruction _____
6. Education information _____
7. Cemetery records _____
8. Important telephone numbers _____
9. Inventory and spare key to safe-deposit box _____
10. Receipts for items under warranty _____
11. Receipts for expensive items _____

TAX
1. Tax receipts
2. Paid bill receipts
   (with deductible receipts filed separately to facilitate tax preparation and possibly reduce taxes)
3. Brokerage transaction advices
4. Income tax working papers
5. Credit statements
6. Income and expense records for rental properties
7. Medical, dental, and drug expenses
8. Records of business expenses

III. ITEMS FOR STORAGE IN HOME INACTIVE FILE

1. Prior tax returns
2. Home improvement records
3. Brokerage advices (prior to three most recent years)
4. Family health records (prior to three most recent years)
5. Proof that major debts or other major contracts have been met
6. Canceled checks (prior to three most recent years)

The major reason for keeping an *inactive file* is to prove past tax returns. This file should contain important papers—formerly stored in your active file—that are over three years old. After six years most people can safely discard their records, although you will want to keep receipts that prove any improvements you have made to your home. You may also want to keep old tax returns as a matter of curiosity—to show your great grandchildren that it was once possible to live on less than $100,000 per year. At the present rate of inflation, they'll probably be earning $100,000 per *month!*

CHECKING THE SYMPTOMS WITH PERSONAL FINANCIAL STATEMENTS

If you operate your own practice, you are well aware of the importance of preparing business financial statements periodically. It is equally important to prepare personal financial statements. Two types of statements should suffice. The first is a statement of personal assets and liabilities, which will summarize your assets, liabilities, and net worth. The second is a personal budget which summarizes where your income comes from and how you spend (or perhaps fritter) it. You don't need an accountant to prepare your personal financial statements, although you do need to pull some records together. If your financial situation is quite complicated, however, you may ask your accountant to assist you in preparing them if you haven't already. A Personal Budget Planner appears in Chapter 3, and a blank Statement of Personal Assets and Liabilities form is included here to help you to summarize your assets and liabilities.

STATEMENT OF PERSONAL ASSETS AND LIABILITIES

A statement of personal assets and liabilities is an excellent way to gauge your progress toward financial security. Be sure to list assets at their current market values, but be realistic when valuing real estate and personal possessions like cars and furniture. If you have a lot of real estate and stock that have appreciated considerably in value, remember that your net worth might not be as high as it seems if you eventually liquidate those assets, since you will have to pay a capital gains tax on them. Finally, be sure to list all liabilities. People have a tendency to understate liabilities.

Once you have prepared an up-to-date balance sheet, you can then make plans to increase your net worth. If you have recently begun your career, don't be dismayed if your net worth is nil or negative. The important thing is to take action to improve it. That's why the Statement of Personal Assets and Liabilities has three columns. You should prepare it every six months so that you can monitor the improvement in your net worth.

STATEMENT OF PERSONAL ASSETS AND LIABILITIES

This work sheet can be used to summarize your assets and liabilities. Three columns are included so that you can periodically monitor your progress. This statement should be prepared at least once per year, and many people prepare it more frequently.

	19____	19____	19____
ASSETS			
1. Cash in checking and brokerage accounts	$_____	$_____	$_____
2. Money market funds and accounts	_____	_____	_____
3. Fixed-income investments:			
■ Savings accounts	_____	_____	_____
■ CDs	_____	_____	_____
■ Government securities and funds	_____	_____	_____
■ Mortgage-backed securities and funds	_____	_____	_____
■ Corporate bonds and bond funds	_____	_____	_____
■ Municipal bonds and bond funds	_____	_____	_____
■ Other fixed-income investments	_____	_____	_____
4. Stock investments:			
■ Common stock in publicly traded companies	_____	_____	_____
■ Stock mutual funds	_____	_____	_____
■ Other stock investments	_____	_____	_____
5. Real estate investments:			
■ Undeveloped land	_____	_____	_____
■ Directly owned, income-producing real estate	_____	_____	_____
■ Real estate limited partnerships	_____	_____	_____
6. Ownership interest in private business	_____	_____	_____

7. Cash value of life insurance
   policies   _____ _____ _____

8. Retirement-oriented assets:
   ■ Individual retirement accounts   _____ _____ _____
   ■ Salary reduction 401(k) plans   _____ _____ _____
   ■ Keogh or simplified employee
     pension plans   _____ _____ _____
   ■ Vested interest in corporate
     pension and profit-sharing
     plans   _____ _____ _____
   ■ Employee thrift and stock-
     purchase plans   _____ _____ _____
   ■ Tax-deferred annuities   _____ _____ _____
   ■ Other retirement-oriented
     assets   _____ _____ _____

9. Personal assets:
   ■ Personal residence(s)   _____ _____ _____
   ■ Automobile(s)   _____ _____ _____
   ■ Jewelry   _____ _____ _____
   ■ Personal property   _____ _____ _____

10. Other assets:
    ■ _____ _____ _____ _____
    ■ _____ _____ _____ _____
    ■ _____ _____ _____ _____
    ■ _____ _____ _____ _____

11. Total assets: $_____ $_____ $_____

LIABILITIES
1. Credit cards and charge
   accounts $_____ $_____ $_____
2. Income taxes payable   _____ _____ _____
3. Miscellaneous accounts
   payable   _____ _____ _____
4. Bank loans   _____ _____ _____
5. Policy loans on life insurance
   policies   _____ _____ _____
6. Automobile loans   _____ _____ _____
7. Student loans   _____ _____ _____
8. Mortgages on personal
   residence(s)   _____ _____ _____

9. Mortgages on investment real
   estate   _____   _____   _____
10. Broker's margin loans   _____   _____   _____
11. Limited partnership debt   _____   _____   _____
12. Other liabilities:
   ■ _____   _____   _____   _____
   ■ _____   _____   _____   _____
   ■ _____   _____   _____   _____
13. Total liabilities: $_____ $_____ $_____
14. Net worth (total assets less
    total liabilities): $_____ $_____ $_____

Note: Assets should be listed at their current market values. Be realistic in valuing those assets that require an estimate of market value, such as your home and personal property.

PERSONAL BUDGET

Budgeting is as important for individuals and families as it is for businesses. The purposes of budgeting are: to define possible problems in the way you spend your money; to identify opportunities to overcome these problems; and to help you plan realistically to improve your spending habits. Knowing both the amount of income that can reasonably be expected and how that income is spent can go far in preventing the duress and domestic squabbles that often result from unforeseen financial burdens. Tips on controlling your spending and preparing a budget appear in Chapter 3.

TAKING CONTROL OF YOUR FINANCIAL FUTURE

Many health-care professionals think that they have neither the knowledge nor the spare time to manage their personal financial affairs effectively. The danger of this perception is that they may end up abdicating responsibility for these matters to others, often with predictably unfortunate results. In order to take control over your financial future, you need to select your investment, insurance, and legal advisers carefully; decide whether or not you need a financial planner; and avoid making bad financial decisions.

SELECTING AND MANAGING YOUR ADVISERS

Busy health-care professionals all too often either fail to select appropriate financial advisers or neglect to manage them effectively. You probably need to take a more active role in making sure your advisers are providing the best possible advice and service. The three most common family advisers are discussed below.

Stockbroker. It is certainly no secret that stockbrokers have an inherent conflict of interest in advising you on your investments. You are usually better off buying and holding, while the broker not only has to generate transactions but also has additional incentive to promote products that his or her firm wants promoted. Nevertheless, there are many excellent stockbrokers who can deal with these conflicts and still act in your best interest. Often, these brokers are those who have established themselves in the business (versus a new broker, who is usually under an inordinate amount of pressure to generate commissions).

Once you have found a good broker, you need to state your investment parameters clearly. Firmly reject any suggested new investments or changes in your portfolio if you feel they are inappropriate. Do not get into the habit of simply consenting to all broker recommendations. Eventually, a good broker will understand your investment approach and a mutually satisfactory relationship will be formed.

Insurance agent. It is usually better to select an independent insurance agent who has the capability and willingness to shop among several carriers for the best possible coverage rather than one who represents a single company. Insurance agents also have a conflict of interest in that certain insurance products pay much higher commissions than other, more mundane products. In the worst of instances, mediocre agents may not even suggest essential coverage to you (umbrella liability insurance, for example) because it provides such a low commission. The better agents will review your coverage with you at least annually and will be willing to shop for appropriate policies. Moreover, effective agents will go to bat for you when necessary. For example, if you are having difficulty securing disability insurance because of a health problem, a good agent will work hard to find the necessary insurance at the best possible price. To assure a good relationship, you must keep the agent informed of changes in your circumstances, and if necessary, insist on a periodic review of your coverage.

Attorney. Many doctors and dentists accumulate sizable estates that require much more than basic estate planning techniques. One of the most important considerations in selecting legal counsel is to find an attorney or a firm that can accommodate what are often increasingly complex legal needs as your estate grows. In other words, the attorney who can handle simple wills and powers of attorney may not be capable of preparing more complex trust documents if and when this need eventually arises. If you do outgrow your attorney's expertise, you must seek more experienced counsel. Beyond that, your attorney should be responsive to your needs and should conduct his or her work in a timely manner.

Finding the right advisers is well worth the effort. There is no ideal way to locate these professionals, but word-of-mouth recommendation can be an important first step. Also, if you're unhappy with one of your advisers, it may be because you have not taken an active role in the relationship. If the problem persists, do not hesitate to make a change. It's amazing how many people dislike or distrust their advisers, yet continue to do business with them.

DO YOU NEED A FINANCIAL PLANNER?

Financial planning is on everyone's mind these days, and several hundred thousand people now call themselves "financial planners." Some work on commission, some strictly on fees, and some collect both commissions and fees. You should expect to pay anywhere from $2,000 to $10,000 for consultations and a comprehensive, truly objective financial plan from a fee-based financial planner. While financial planning sounds like a service everyone could use, many people do not benefit significantly. One reason for this is that most financial planners are simply not capable of dealing with the multiplicity of matters that affect your financial well-being, including insurance, investments, credit management, pensions, and estate planning.

Some medical professionals, typically those with high incomes or high net worths, can certainly benefit from the process, but I am a firm believer that many people can and should do their own financial planning. It requires a modest amount of reading and research, combined with periodic reviews of family finances, much as described in this book. Incidentally, the whole process can be fun. Those who feel that they need a financial planner—perhaps for a particular problem, rather than a comprehensive review—obviously have many to choose from. If you need to be assured of objectivity, consider selecting a CPA or estate planning attorney who is committed to the financial planning process. As with all of your advisers, word-of-mouth recommendation is a good way to find competent financial planners.

AVOIDING MISTAKES

Whether you rely heavily on financial advisers or not, you typically have to make a variety of decisions that will, hopefully, enhance your well-being. Unfortunately, the road to financial security contains many potholes that can slow your progress, sometimes significantly. Just as the investment homily advises, "The best way to win in the stock market is by not losing," in financial planning the best way to achieve financial security is by avoiding mistakes. Listed below are ten common errors that many doctors, nurses, and other health-care professionals make in the course of trying to improve their financial status.

1. *Neglecting to cover gaps in insurance coverage.* The surest way to wipe out years of hard-earned accumulation of capital is to suffer an uninsured loss. Doctors and dentists usually have abundant professional liability insurance, but they often have shortcomings in other areas, particularly long-term disability insurance and life insurance. Deficiencies in any area of insurance can be disastrous. This is why insurance is covered early in this book (see Chapter 2).

2. *Making dumb investments.* Everyone gets duped into making inappropriate investments at least once in his or her lifetime. Unfortunately, many doctors, dentists, and other highly compensated health-care professionals make more than their share.

3. *Utilizing inappropriate strategies.* While there are numerous very complex financial strategies available to anyone who wants to use them, they often make little or no sense. Many are

---

At the present rate of growth in the financial planning profession, by the year 2000 every man, woman, and child over the age of three in the United States will be a "financial planner."

tax motivated, and well-to-do doctors and dentists are very receptive as a result. For example, many advisers urge wealthy parents to give money to their children in order to take advantage of their lower income-tax bracket. On the surface, this sounds like a great deal. The money is eventually going to pay college tuition anyway, so why not save tax dollars along the way? Well, the tax savings really aren't that great, and worse, this strategy could end up backfiring. For most families, transferring $25,000 to a child over the age of thirteen will end up saving less than $300 in federal income taxes each year. Big deal. If the child is age thirteen or less, the tax savings will be even less. Worse, by shifting money to a child, many families end up qualifying for less financial aid than they would have, had the money remained in the parents' name.

4. *Shifting investments too often.* Why do so many investors change their investments at the slightest provocation? Many medical professionals have the wherewithal (meaning cash) to react to any new investment fad that comes along. Alas, the results are predictable.

5. *Failing to plan ahead for tax minimization.* Most people wait until December to begin planning to minimize taxes for the current year. While current tax rules have eliminated many tax-reduction techniques, opportunities still exist, and just as before, they require advance planning—years of advance planning in some instances.

6. *Failing to take full advantage of the many tax breaks available to the self-employed.* Uncle Sam offers numerous tax breaks to self-employed people, which, unfortunately, too many self-employed health-care professionals fail to take advantage of.

7. *Failing to accumulate sufficient retirement resources.* Because of their long and expensive period of training, doctors and dentists have fewer years in which to accumulate sufficient resources to fund a comfortable retirement. This, combined with financial pressures on the health-care system, may prevent many health-care professionals from accumulating sufficient resources to assure a comfortable retirement—unless they recognize these matters and begin to address them.

8. *Neglecting to take full advantage of appropriate estate planning techniques.* Many medical professionals accumulate sizable estates—often in spite of their spending habits and lackluster investment results. The owner of the estate and his or her heirs can benefit both before and after death from any of a number of useful, but not well known, estate planning techniques.

9. *Giving up control to financial advisers.* As mentioned at the beginning of this section, many doctors and dentists make the mistake of abdicating responsibility for handling their money and financial affairs, deferring to various advisers. Although it is often appropriate to rely on the expertise of competent advisers, by not taking an active role in personal financial matters, they will simply not receive the level of service they need and deserve.

10. *Failing to adjust to the new realities of the health-care business.* Many health-care experts are predicting that medical professionals will have to look forward to a long period of belt tightening in the health-care system. This may well translate into lower compensation, or at the very least, a dampening effect on salary increases. Further, fringe benefits, including pension plans, are likely to be reduced. Perhaps it's wishful thinking, but many health-care professionals are not yet adjusting or even planning to adjust their personal finances to reflect the new realities.

No one can avoid making mistakes in their personal financial planning. Some people, however, make too many mistakes, and worse, repeat them. As you review the above list, identify areas where you need improvement and pay close attention when they are addressed later in this book. The following Financial Planning and Record-Keeping Action Plan will help you keep track of which steps you've dealt with successfully and which still require your attention. This action plan, as well as the ones that appear at the end of each chapter, should be reviewed periodically to remain useful. Space is provided at the end of each action plan to make comments and to list important items that you need to focus on.

FINANCIAL PLANNING AND RECORD-KEEPING ACTION PLAN

Current Status		
Needs Action	Okay or Not Applicable	
☐	☐	1. Set some realistic financial planning goals, and plan how you are going to achieve them.
☐	☐	2. If you experience any major changes in your personal or financial status, review how your new circumstances will affect your overall financial planning.
☐	☐	3. Discuss money matters openly and regularly with your partner.
☐	☐	4. Create a personal record-keeping system that is comprehensive enough to be useful yet is simple enough that you will use it.
☐	☐	5. Prepare a statement of personal assets and liabilities periodically to measure your financial planning progress.
☐	☐	6. Select your financial advisers with care, and be aware of any potential conflicts of interest that they might have.
☐	☐	7. If you are not satisfied with any of your financial advisers, don't hesitate to make a change.
☐	☐	8. Be particularly careful in selecting a financial planner. Be sure he or she has the qualifications that are necessary to meet your needs.

Current Status

Needs Action	Okay or Not Applicable	
☐	☐	9. Of the ten common mistakes that health-care professionals make (listed at the end of this chapter), list those that represent potential problems in your situation:

_____

_____

_____

_____

_____

_____

Comments: _____

_____

_____

_____

_____

Financial Planning and Record-Keeping "To Do" List: _____

_____

_____

_____

_____

Now that you've established your objectives, organized your records, and determined where you stand financially, you're ready to start taking charge of your financial life. The first matter to discuss is insurance, because without appropriate insurance coverage, everything else in your financial planning life is in jeopardy.

The key to achieving riches beyond your wildest imagination: Never own anything that eats.

2 Insurance: Financial Preventive Medicine

You may be tempted to skip this chapter, thinking there is nothing more boring than insurance. But if you are so inclined, you might as well skip the rest of the book, because unless you have adequate insurance coverage, there is no sense in doing the more exciting things associated with personal financial planning, like investing and planning for a financially comfortable retirement. The reason for this is that a single gap in your insurance coverage could jeopardize a lifetime's worth of sacrifice and savings. So, adequate insurance coverage is every bit as important in planning for your financial security as the other, more appealing personal financial matters.

AVOIDING MISTAKES IN INSURANCE COVERAGE

Most people understand the need for health insurance, life insurance, homeowner's insurance, and automobile insurance, yet they often leave gaps in their coverage that could prove to be very costly. Although many people are aware of how devastating the loss of assets or earning power can be to themselves and their families, only a few take well thought out, informed steps to insure themselves against that possibility. While your insurance agent can be indispensable in helping you obtain and maintain adequate coverage, you probably need to take more control over the process.

Insurance products are becoming increasingly sophisticated

and differentiated. While the level of confusion surrounding insurance is just getting worse, many of the new insurance products on the market are better.

In order to avoid making mistakes in securing adequate insurance coverage, you must keep the following in mind.

COVER ALL GAPS

You and your insurance agent must be sure that all foreseeable areas of risk are covered with insurance. The most common gaps in coverage are lack of an umbrella liability policy (often called extended liability insurance), inadequate long-term disability coverage (particularly if you are self-employed), and insufficient coverage on valuable personal possessions, such as jewelry and silverware.

OBTAIN THE CORRECT POLICY COVERAGE

Each of the policies that you need to purchase must be evaluated in detail so that you are assured of receiving the coverage you need. As you will find from the discussion later in this chapter, policies can vary significantly as to extent of coverage they offer. This does not necessarily mean you need to purchase the most comprehensive policy, but you need to ensure that the coverage meets your needs. Policy limits are also an important consideration. For example, an otherwise excellent health policy might have a major-medical cap that is too low.

ADJUST COVERAGE TO MEET YOUR CHANGING NEEDS

Even though you may have adequate coverage now, your needs will undoubtedly change in the future. Therefore, you need to review the adequacy of your insurance coverage at least annually, and if there is an obvious change in your status, such as the birth of a child or a job change, you need an immediate review.

MINIMIZE THE COST OF INSURANCE

Many segments of the insurance industry are intensely competitive, and premiums for similar policy coverage can vary dramatically. You may well be able to achieve significant savings

TABLE   2

Important Areas of Insurance Coverage

TYPE OF INSURANCE	DESCRIPTION/FEATURES
Health Insurance	Protects you from both the out-of-pocket costs of health care and large cash outflows during major illness.
Homeowner's Insurance	Property, such as a home, other structures, personal property, and general contents of the dwelling are insured against theft or destruction; protects against the possibility of cash outflows for replacement of these assets.
Renter's Insurance	Protects the personal possessions of the tenant.
Automobile Insurance	Protects you from large cash outflows for damages resulting from automobile accident or theft.
Personal Liability Insurance	Protects you from having personal assets or future earnings forfeited as a result of a personal liability suit. Provides additional protection on top of homeowner's and automobile liability coverage.
Professional Liability Insurance	Protects you from claims arising out of professional acts or omissions.
Disability Insurance	Replaces part or most of your wage income in the event of disability.
Life Insurance	Replaces part or most of your wage income in the event of your death and covers nonrecurring expenses of your dependents during a readjustment period after death.

with careful shopping and selection of policy features. Cheaper does not necessarily mean better, but studies have shown that many people pay far more for their insurance coverage than they need to.

While securing the right kind of insurance coverage does not vary significantly from occupation to occupation, many health-care professionals do have unique needs that must be addressed in order to ensure that their coverage is comprehensive.

■ Professional liability insurance is essential for most health-care professionals, unless it is already provided by your employer. This coverage is often costly, and some practitioners are removing assets from their estates in order to reduce or eliminate the need for medical malpractice insurance. This strategy will be covered later on in this chapter.

■ Many health-care professionals have insufficient disability income insurance coverage, particularly if they are self-employed. This coverage is expensive and, therefore, employers often do not provide sufficient coverage to meet the needs of higher income health-care workers. High cost also discourages many self-employed medical practitioners from obtaining adequate disability insurance.

■ High-income professionals often fail to obtain enough life insurance to enable their dependents to sustain a standard of living that is equivalent to their living standard when the insured was alive.

■ Because of their wealth and prominence in the community, many doctors and dentists need higher limits of insurance coverage than might otherwise be necessary. For example, doctors should often have high-limit umbrella liability insurance because, sadly, they represent attractive targets for personal liability lawsuits.

Why do they call it "life" insurance when you have to die in order to collect on the policy?

■ Because of the demands on their time, many health-care professionals rely too heavily on their insurance agent or their financial adviser to evaluate and obtain insurance coverage. This can result not only in securing inappropriate coverage, but also paying too much for it.

The following sections will provide some guidance on selecting appropriate and comprehensive insurance. The table summarizes the major areas of insurance coverage.

LIFE INSURANCE

Although the primary goal of life insurance is to provide adequate resources for the deceased's dependents, it can also provide for other postmortem financial needs, including paying estate taxes and assuring that a professional practice will continue to operate or can be sold in an orderly fashion. If you are confused about the complexities involved in selecting life insurance, you are not alone. This is an industry that seems to thrive on obfuscation.

ESTIMATING YOUR LIFE INSURANCE NEEDS

Figuring out how much life insurance you need is no easy task. Most of us are either underinsured or overinsured. Of course, the people who need a lot of life insurance are those who have dependent children. But children are not necessarily the only dependents you might have. For example, "dinks," or dual-income couples with no kids may need more life insurance than they think if, as is often the case, they are enjoying a life-style that is so profligate that a surviving spouse would be financially crippled by the other's demise. You probably know some dinks— they often have a huge mortgage, ever-present car loans, and no savings.

If you are concerned about providing for dependents, one way to estimate your insurance needs is to look at two extremes— a maximum and a minimum. First, figure out how much insurance it would take to provide for all of your dependents' financial needs. This would typically include payment of readjustment expenses during the period immediately after your demise, plus paying off your outstanding debts, plus income for your spouse throughout his or her lifetime. Obviously, if you buy enough insurance to cover all expenses, your spouse will undoubtedly be the most financially desirable widow or widower in town. So the other extreme you need to estimate is a minimum amount that will allow your family a few years to become self-sufficient after your death. This may be an amount equivalent to four or five years of your net income—enough to allow your family some time to get back on a firm economic footing. If you can estimate the extremes, you can then make a sensible decision as to an amount that is appropriate for you and your dependents. The following Life Insurance Needs Work Sheet will help you make this decision.

LIFE INSURANCE NEEDS WORK SHEET

This work sheet can be used to estimate your life insurance needs.

If you enter amounts for each category of need, the resulting estimate should be viewed as a *maximum* amount of insurance that will meet all foreseeable needs of your survivors.

Note: All amounts should be expressed in terms of current dollars.

EXPENSES
 1. Final expenses (one-time expenses incurred by your death)
   a. Final illness (medical costs will probably exceed health insurance deductibles and coinsurance, so assume you will have to fund at least those amounts) $...........
   b. Burial/funeral costs   ....
   c. Probate costs (if unsure, assume 4 percent of assets passing through the probate process)   ....
   d. Federal estate taxes (for most estates over $600,000 willed to someone other than spouse)   ....
   e. State inheritance taxes (varies by state)   ....
   f. Legal fees, estate administration   ....
   g. Other   ....
   h. Total final expenses $...........
 2. Outstanding debt (to be paid off at your death)
   a. Credit card/consumer debt   ....
   b. Car   ....
   c. Mortgage (if it's to be paid off at your death; otherwise, include payments in life income)   ....
   d. Other   ....
   e. Total outstanding debt $...........
 3. Readjustment expenses (to cover the transition period of immediate crisis)

a. Child care ....
b. Additional homemaking help ....
c. Vocational counseling/educational training
   (for a nonworking or underemployed
   spouse who expects to seek paid
   employment) ....
d. Other ....
e. Total readjustment expenses $............
4. Dependency expenses (until all children are self-supporting)
   a. Estimate all your household's current
      annual expenditures ....
   b. To remove the deceased person's
      expenses, multiply this figure by:
      .70 for a surviving family of one
      .74 for a surviving family of two
      .78 for a surviving family of three
      .80 for a surviving family of four
      .82 for a surviving family of five
      $..... (Line 4a) × ..... (factor) = ...
   c. Deduct spouse's estimated annual
      income from employment (.......)
   d. Equals current annual expenses to be
      covered by currently owned assets and
      insurance ....
   e. To determine approximate total
      dependency expenses required, multiply
      by number of years until youngest child
      becomes self-supporting:
      $..... (Line 4b) x ..... (years) = ...
   f. If support for dependent parent(s) is to be
      provided, multiply annual support by the
      number of years such support is expected
      to continue: $....... × ..... (years) = ...
   g. Total dependency expenses (add Lines 4e
      and 4f) $............
5. Education expenses
   a. Annual private school tuition in
      current dollars (if desired) ....
   b. Multiply by number of years and children
      left to attend:
      $....... (Line 5a) × ..... (years) = ...
   c. Annual college costs in current
      dollars ....
   d. Multiply by number of years and children
      left to attend:
      $....... (Line 5c) × ..... (years) = ...
   e. Total education expenses (add Lines 5b
      and 5d) $............

6. Life income (for the surviving spouse after the children are all self-supporting)
   a. Annual amount desired (in current dollars) ....
   b. Deduct spouse's estimated annual income from employment (.......)
   c. Equals annual expenses to be covered by currently owned assets and insurance ....
   d. Multiply by number of years between when the youngest child becomes self-supporting and the surviving spouse begins receiving Social Security benefits and other retirement income, if any:
      $....... (Line 6c) × ..... (years) = $..........
7. Retirement income for surviving spouse
   a. Annual amount desired in current dollars (less Social Security and any pension income) ....
   b. Multiply by number of years of life expectancy after retirement begins:
      $....... (Line 7a) × ..... (years) = $..........
8. Total funds needed to cover expenses: (add Lines 1h, 2e, 3e, 4g, 5e, 6d, and 7b) $..........

ASSETS CURRENTLY AVAILABLE TO SUPPORT FAMILY
   Proceeds from life insurance already owned $..........
   Cash and savings   ....
   Equity in real estate (if survivors will sell)   ....
   Securities   ....
   IRA and Keogh plans   ....
   Employer savings plans   ....
   Lump-sum employer pension benefits   ....
   Other sources   ....
9. Total assets $..........

ADDITIONAL LIFE INSURANCE REQUIRED
10. Subtract available assets (Line 9) from total funds needed to cover expenses (Line 8).
    This shortfall represents the estimated amount that must be covered through life insurance. $..........

Your life insurance needs typically decline as you age. In order to plan the kind of insurance that you need, you should not only estimate how much coverage you need now but also how much you expect to need in the future. Finally, don't rely too much on someone else's estimate of your life insurance requirements. The insurance industry loves to run projections for potential policyholders, and these projections can be very helpful. But as we all understand, the insurance company estimates are not likely to err on the low side when it comes to estimating how much life insurance you need.

If you have your own practice or are a member of a group practice, you may need to consider the use of life insurance to assure an orderly disposition of your business interest as well as to assure that your survivors are compensated adequately for your interest. Such arrangements are called *buy-sell agreements*, and are often funded with life insurance policies. Working out the details of these arrangements requires the combined expertise of your attorney, accountant, and insurance adviser.

Many health-care professionals manage to amass large estates. If you are either beginning your career or just now emerging from the impoverishment that often results from the cost of your education, training, or the cost of establishing a practice, you probably can't envision accumulating an estate that would incur substantial estate taxes. Nevertheless, you may eventually be in that position. Therefore, you should at least consider using life insurance to assist in paying off your estate taxes when the time comes, because if your estate lacks sufficient cash or assets that are readily convertible into cash, your survivors may have to liquidate valuable and productive assets to pay death taxes and administrative expenses. Careful planning is necessary, of course, and your advisers may well recommend that you establish an *irrevocable life insurance trust* as the best means of providing estate liquidity. If you are married with children, you should probably consider a so-called "second to die" life insurance policy. This policy would name you and your spouse as joint insureds, and pays the death benefit only at the death of the second spouse. Second-to-die policies offer lower premiums and make sense in many instances since no federal estate tax is incurred upon the death of the first spouse, owing to the unlimited marital deduction.

WHAT KIND OF LIFE INSURANCE POLICIES ARE RIGHT FOR YOU?

Once you have an idea of how much life insurance you need, you must then try to figure out the best kind of coverage to obtain, if any, in addition to the coverage you undoubtedly already have. The following table summarizes the various types of life insurance products.

Life Insurance Policy Alternatives

TYPE OF POLICY	DESCRIPTION/FEATURES
Term	Term insurance only provides death protection. A term policy does not build a cash value. If the insured discontinues insurance premium payments, the coverage simply lapses after a specific grace period. This is the cheapest form of immediate insurance protection. There are many kinds of term insurance. Term insurance premiums increase with age, for the same amount of coverage, although most people's life insurance requirements decrease with age. A *renewable term* policy covers the insured for a fixed period of years or until a specified age. With renewable term, the insured may usually renew the policy each year without a medical examination. *Decreasing term* provides constant premiums over time with a declining amount of death protection.
Whole Life	Also called *straight* or *ordinary life.* Requires level premium payments over the lifetime of the insured and provides cash value, which increases slowly in the early years and more rapidly in the later years of the policy. The rate of increase in the cash value is predetermined. A variety of variations are also available. Under a *limited payment life* policy, premium payments remain level up to a certain age and then cease. *Adjustable life* plans allow the insured to change both the premium payments and the face amount of the policy as needs and income vary.
Universal Life	*Universal life* permits flexible premium payments. The cash value portion of the policy is deposited into an interest-bearing account that is usually tied to a

TYPE OF POLICY	DESCRIPTION/FEATURES
	predetermined index. Most universal policies allow the insured to increase the death protection, although another medical examination may be required. Universal life insurance policies have been designed to provide considerable flexibility to the amount of coverage and the amount of premium.
Variable Life	The cash value portion of *variable life* is invested in one or more stock, bond, and money market funds of the policyholder's choosing. Therefore, the cash value will fluctuate based on the performance of these separate investment accounts.
Single Premium Whole Life	*Single premium* policies are paid up in one or very few installments. The emphasis in these policies is on investment, not insurance. Like other cash value policies, the cash values build up tax free.

CASH VALUE OR TERM?

Life insurance is a commodity item in an intensely competitive industry. While most life insurance is sold, not purchased, you may benefit from comparison shopping for the lowest-priced policy that meets your needs. Whether term insurance or cash value is the preferable method is, has been, and always will be the subject of intense debate. Most financial planning matters need not be reduced to an either/or decision. This can be said of the term vs. cash value insurance dilemma. The decision depends upon your individual circumstance, but many health-care professionals who enjoy a high income and require considerable life insurance may benefit from a combination of term insurance and *some* cash value insurance. You should not attempt to meet all of your life insurance needs through cash value coverage, because of the high premiums associated with cash value insurance. I have found that many doctors and dentists have too much cash value insurance. While the tax-deferral features are certainly attractive, the generally high commissions and fees associated with these policies drag down returns in comparison with returns that can be garnered on other investments.

If you find that you need more term insurance, there are several sources of low-cost coverage you should investigate. First, you might want to check with your employer to see if you can add, at your own expense, to the life insurance that is already provided by your employer. If you happen to be self-employed, you may be able to arrange for increased life insurance through your group carrier. The rates are usually very attractive. Another source of low-cost insurance coverage is through professional groups and associations. Numerous associations for health-care professionals offer very attractive rates to their members. Coverage is also available to spouses through these group insurance programs.

You may be unhappy with a cash value policy that you have already purchased, probably because you didn't understand it when it was sold to you, and upon reflection you realize that it is an expensive way to buy life insurance protection, and the cash value side of the policy isn't such a hot investment. Should you cash the policy in? Probably not, particularly if you've been paying premiums on it for a number of years, because the cash-value increase will become more attractive as the policy ages. Since most of your initial premiums went to pay commissions and other fees, you probably shouldn't cash in a relatively new policy either.

ADDITIONAL TIPS FOR SECURING APPROPRIATE LIFE COVERAGE

Make sure your term insurance policies are *renewable*, which guarantees that you will be able to renew your policy for an additional term, albeit at a higher annual premium. Incidentally, a lender may encourage you to purchase *decreasing term* when you take out a mortgage, automobile, or other installment loan. The amount of insurance coverage decreases over time as your outstanding loan balance decreases. If you think decreasing term is a good idea for a large loan, you're probably better off shopping around for coverage, since the policies offered by lending institutions are usually expensive—as much as twenty times more expensive than comparable group policies!

If you are turned down for life insurance due to a health condition, don't despair. A good agent will find coverage for you, and you'll probably be surprised at how little additional premium is required, if any. If your agent can't help you, some insurance agencies have specialists in substandard risks. You also might be able to find a nonmedical group policy.

Affluent medical professionals must be particularly careful when specifying policy owners and beneficiaries. These designations can have significant estate planning implications, and the earlier you resolve these matters, the better. Don't rely on your agent to advise you; use a good estate planning attorney instead. Remember, while the proceeds of your life insurance policy are not subject to income taxes (the agents love to tell you this), they may be subject to estate taxes (funny, they don't tell you this). There are ways around this, but like all other sophisticated estate planning techniques, they require considerable legal expertise.

HEALTH INSURANCE

You need not be reminded of the importance of adequate and continuous medical insurance. But you do need to be aware that policies vary in what they do and do not cover. Whether you are an employee of a health-care institution or are self-employed, the rapidly escalating cost of health insurance means you are probably going to be required either to pay more for coverage or accept reduced coverage. Either way, you must plan carefully to meet all foreseeable expenses, particularly if they are going to come out of your own pocket. If your major medical policy has an upper limit of coverage that makes you uncomfortable, you may want to consider purchasing an excess major medical policy separately. This coverage is relatively inexpensive.

If you are self-employed, you are probably becoming aware of the difficulty experienced by small businesses to obtain adequate medical coverage at a reasonable cost. Like any of the other insurance coverage areas, you or your insurance adviser will benefit from investigating the policies offered by several carriers. Also, you should consider the group medical insurance coverage at more attractive group rates. Alternatively, you may want to consider an individually purchased major medical policy with a high deductible if you can afford the amount of the deductible comfortably.

> If I bought the amount of life insurance my agent tells me I need, my wife would not only be able to buy the nicest plot in the town cemetery to bury me; she'd also be able to buy the whole town.

A few other health insurance considerations may also apply to you. Be sure that your children always have sufficient medical coverage, even if they have left the nest and are on their own. If your children are in college, be sure that your policy covers them adequately, and if not, don't expect the group plan offered by your child's college to be adequate.

If your parents are retired, check with them to make sure that they have Medicare Gap insurance to supplement Medicare. Also, make sure they don't fall prey to unscrupulous agents who attempt to sell them either duplicative policies or narrowly defined insurance policies, like cancer insurance.

Finally, if you are traveling overseas, make sure your medical insurance carrier will provide coverage. Most do. Medicare, however, does not provide any coverage outside the United States (except in Canada and Mexico, under very limited circumstances). Therefore, Medicare-eligible travelers should purchase a medical policy that will cover them during their sojourn abroad. These low-cost policies are available through travel agencies.

DISABILITY INSURANCE

Although the insurance industry seems most concerned about selling life insurance, you are far more likely to suffer from a long-term disability during your working years than you are to die. Long-term disability coverage is, therefore, essential unless you are fortunate to have sufficient resources to support yourself even if you can't work. Yet many health-care professionals, particularly those who are self-employed, don't realize that their coverage is either insufficient in amount or lacking important policy provisions. If you have your own practice, it is particularly crucial for you to have your own comprehensive disability insurance.

DETERMINING HOW MUCH YOU NEED

Many people whose employers provide long-term disability coverage think that this coverage is sufficient. That may or may

---

It's okay not to have any health insurance—just don't get sick.

not be the case. A short-term disability resulting from, say, a heart attack, arthritis, or an accident can seriously disrupt one's financial life. A long-term disability is certain to be financially, emotionally, and professionally traumatic. With adequate disability insurance coverage, you can at least minimize your financial loss. The following work sheet will allow you to estimate approximately how much additional disability insurance coverage you need.

One other matter that bears on your estimate of the amount of disability insurance you need is the taxability of benefits. Disability income is taxable if payments are attributable to employer contributions to a disability plan. Benefits are excludable from income if you, rather than your employer, make contributions to the plan. Therefore, if you are an employee, you may want to consider paying your own disability insurance premium rather than having your employer make it. Sure, this costs you more, but it may be worth it in exchange for your being able to receive the disability payments tax free, should you ever become disabled.

DISABILITY INCOME NEEDS WORK SHEET

Resources needed:
1. Total annual family living expenses $........
2. Subtract annual expenses that would go away if you became disabled, such as taxes (disability benefits may be partly or fully tax free), work-related expenses, entertainment, and travel (.......)
3. Adjusted annual family living expenses
   (subtract Line 2 from Line 1)   ....

Resources available:
4. Annual income from savings and investments
   (dividends and interest)   ....
5. Annual income from spouse's job   ....
6. Annual disability benefits provided by employer's policy   ....
7. Annual disability benefits provided by other disability policies
   currently owned   ....
8. Total available resources
   (add Lines 4, 5, 6, and 7)   ....
9. Additional resources needed either from liquidating assets or
   additional disability insurance (subtract Line 8 from Line 3) $........

WHERE TO OBTAIN COVERAGE

Disability coverage offered by health-care employers varies widely in policy limits and features. Some are quite good, but others are unsatisfactory. You can understand why so many group policies offer limited benefits, if you are self-employed and have obtained coverage for yourself and your employees. Good disability insurance is expensive, even on a group basis. Yet group coverage is considerably cheaper than individually purchased policies. Many professional groups and associations offer lower-cost disability insurance, so you should investigate them if you need more insurance.

Even though you may have access to group disability insurance, you should still consider individually purchased coverage as well, because many of the desirable policy features that are discussed below probably won't be available in a group policy. Disability insurance is nothing to scrimp on. You are seven times more likely to become disabled before you retire than you are to die. If you are a highly compensated physician or dentist and inquire about a large disability policy, be sure to be near some oxygen when you are quoted a price. You may end up paying several thousand dollars per year to obtain good coverage. I think it is money well spent. If you have any health problems, disability insurance will be difficult to obtain, but diligent shopping by an agent who is willing to go to bat for you should get you the coverage you need. Incidentally, the aggregate amount of disability coverage you can receive from all policies, group and individual, generally cannot exceed 80 percent of your earned income, and possibly somewhat less.

IMPORTANT POLICY FEATURES

Disability policies have more features than pharmacies have pills. In addition to guaranteed renewability and noncancellation, the following options and features are well worth considering, if you need to obtain more disability insurance. You might also check the policy features on insurance you already have, both group and individual, against the following. It should help you assess the quality of your existing policies.

It's okay not to have enough disability insurance—just don't become disabled.

DEFINITION OF "DISABILITY"

The best policies will continue disability payments as long as the insured suffers a loss of income. The next level makes payments as long as the insured is unable to perform the "usual and customary" duties of the insured's occupation. Some policies tighten the requirements, defining disability as the inability to perform *all* of the duties of the insured's occupation. This distinction is crucial, for example, in the case of a surgeon whose income was more than $200,000 a year but earns $75,000 as a medical consultant because of blindness. Under the more stringent definition, he would not be entitled to disability payments. Other policies regard disability as the inability to perform any job. You should also check on the policy provisions regarding payments for rehabilitation. Some are very generous, and this is to your advantage, of course.

PERIOD OF COVERAGE

All long-term disability policies have a waiting period between the onset of disability and the date the payments begin. If you are purchasing a policy, lengthening the waiting period will reduce the premium, sometimes considerably. Be sure to get quotes on longer waiting periods—three months, six months, and one year. Benefits should always be payable until age sixty-five, when retirement benefits will presumably kick in.

COST-OF-LIVING ADJUSTMENTS

COLAs are an expensive option, yet they are well worth considering. Most policies pay a fixed monthly benefit as long as you are disabled. The benefit may seem satisfactory now, but would it be ten or twenty years hence, if you become permanently disabled?

PROPERTY INSURANCE

Most people have insurance on their home(s) and automobile(s). Surprisingly, less than one quarter of renters have renter's insurance, although every renter should. Property insurance is pretty straightforward, except that many people fail to understand the limitations of the standard property insurance policy. You need to focus on the commonly overlooked areas of risk in order to assure that you don't have any unpleasant surprises if and when you suffer a loss.

TOTING UP YOUR WORLDLY GOODS

If you come home from work next week and find the fire department shoveling what's left of your home into the back of a truck, could you give your insurer a detailed list of your personal property? If you're like most people, you couldn't even prepare a very complete list of the contents of your wallet, much less the contents of your home. You need to take an inventory of your household possessions. (And you might as well make a list of your wallet contents too.)

A household inventory involves recording pertinent information on your possessions; and the more valuable the possession, the more detailed should be the information. You can do this in writing or by speaking into a tape recorder. Also, take a lot of photographs of your possessions. If you have extensive personal property, you can hire a bonded videotaping service to do the dirty work. Store the inventory information at the office or in your safe-deposit box. Next time you go to the safe-deposit box, make a list of its contents too. When you acquire additional possessions, put the receipts in with your inventory. If you ever suffer a loss, you'll be very glad you have an up-to-date household inventory.

ASSURING COMPLETE COVERAGE

Even if you select comprehensive basic homeowner's and auto policies, you probably haven't covered all the risks that you want to protect against. You probably need some "optional extras" to obtain the coverage you need.

REPLACEMENT COST COVERAGE

Homeowner's insurance should cover 80 to 100 percent of the replacement value of the home, including any improvements that have been made, allowing for annual inflation. The basic insurance coverage usually specifies actual cash value or market value. Using these estimates can lead to underinsurance, however, since repair costs rise faster than the market value of the house. Make sure your policy has sufficient coverage to pay for the total replacement of your home.

Replacement cost coverage on the contents of the house—or in the case of a tenant, the apartment—is usually an extremely valuable option as well. Otherwise, you will be paid actual cash (i.e., depreciated) value for any losses. Not only does this often lead to disputes with the carrier, but it also can result in your having to pay a lot of money out of your own pocket to replace the lost or damaged items. Replacement cost coverage on personal property is normally available as a separate policy rider.

FLOATER POLICIES

Basic homeowner's and renter's policies impose severe limits on the amount they will pay for valuables. Therefore, your valuables should be professionally appraised and covered under a floater. A floater provides a specific amount of insurance for each object on an itemized basis, guaranteeing full replacement value and eliminating deductibles. Floaters should provide "all-risk" coverage—in other words, they will pay no matter what happens to the valuable, even if you unwittingly lose it. Valuables should be reappraised every few years, and floater coverage should be adjusted accordingly. In lieu of a floater policy, you might be able to increase the blanket valuables coverage on your homeowner's or renter's policy from the standard $1,000 to a higher level.

If you store any valuables in a safe-deposit box, you should also obtain a floater that covers these items, since banks rarely insure against loss from safe-deposit boxes.

HOME OFFICE RIDER

Homeowner's insurance does not cover property damage related to the operation of a full- or part-time business in the home. For example, a personal computer within the home that is used primarily for business is not covered. With some exceptions, home office coverage is available as a rider to the basic policy. If a home office rider is not sufficient, a home office policy, available separately, should be obtained.

AUTOMOBILE INSURANCE

Many people pay more for car insurance than they need to. When your policy comes up for renewal, don't just continue the same coverage. Look for ways to save. Higher deductibles, driving a more conservative car, and dropping expensive policy options can result in lower premiums.

PROFESSIONAL AND PERSONAL LIABILITY INSURANCE

OUT, OUT, DAMNED PLAINTIFF'S ATTORNEY!

Professional liability insurance is on the one hand essential for physicians, dentists, and many other health-care professionals, and on the other hand, is becoming prohibitively expensive for some specialties and in some locales. To make matters worse, insurers have been attempting to limit their exposure to loss. If you are in private practice, you are painfully aware of the need for this coverage. If you are an employee of a health-care institution or if you practice both as an employee and on your own, you need to be certain that you are not exposed to any uninsured professional risks.

Most medical liability policies cover *only* liability arising out of professional acts or omissions. The insured's liability as owner or executive officer of a practice may be excluded.

Troubled by the increasing costs of medical liability insurance and threats of litigation, some health-care professionals have taken action to shield their personal assets from potential lawsuits. Methods that have been utilized include incorporation, transferring title to personal assets to a spouse or other relative, and transferring property to an irrevocable trust. The latter two methods render the doctor "penniless." Legal counsel is necessary before any of these alternatives is undertaken.

The most extreme example of adherence to the Hippocratic Oath: performing lifesaving surgery on an uninsured medical malpractice plaintiff's attorney.

DON'T LEAVE HOME WITHOUT YOUR UMBRELLA

Umbrella insurance, also called extended personal liability insurance, is one of the most often overlooked gaps in insurance coverage. If you don't have this coverage, you are jeopardizing assets you currently own and perhaps even some of your future earnings. Similar to the medical malpractice fiasco and spurred on by higher and higher awards in court actions, injured parties, real or fancied, have become more willing to press claims against others for individual acts. If the defendant's assets are insufficient to pay the settlement, the court may award the plaintiff a portion of the defendant's future earnings. I once met a surgeon who told me he had been paying a fortune for professional liability insurance; but he wasn't aware of the need for umbrella coverage until he rear-ended a car driven by a person who, according to the surgeon, made his living jamming on his brakes in front of expensive cars. The surgeon ended up losing a lot of assets and a portion of his future earnings.

INSURANCE COVERAGE CHECKUP
Date: _____

Type of Insurance	Source of Coverage	Check One		
		Coverage Is Adequate	Additional or Improved Coverage Is Necessary	Coverage Is Not Needed
Life	_____	☐	☐	☐
Medical	_____	☐	☐	☐
Disability	_____	☐	☐	☐
Homeowner's/ Renter's	_____	☐	☐	☐
Automobile	_____	☐	☐	☐
Personal Liability (Umbrella)	_____	☐	☐	☐
Professional Liability	_____	☐	☐	☐

Comments _____
_____
_____
_____
_____

Umbrella policies typically protect you and your family (including children away at college and pets) from claims arising out of your nonprofessional activities, including legal defense costs. However, it is important to understand the exclusions written into the umbrella policy.

This coverage is relatively inexpensive; annual premiums for $1,000,000 in liability insurance generally are between $100 and $200. If you are a successful medical professional, $1,000,000 in coverage is probably too little, and some insurers offer up to $10,000,000 in coverage. Umbrella insurance is coordinated with your automobile and homeowner's/renter's insurance policies, so you may have to increase the liability limits on these policies before qualifying for the umbrella. Umbrella insurance is crucial for everyone.

THE CARE AND FEEDING OF INSURANCE AGENTS

A good insurance professional can be a great help in assuring that you are insured adequately and economically. The insurance needs of many health-care professionals are particularly complex, and therefore, the expertise of competent insurance representatives is required. The good ones know their business and know your circumstances. Make them earn their commissions. I'm often asked how you can tell a good agent from a mediocre one. A good agent will review your coverage annually, and will not simply use that occasion to try to sell annuities, mutual funds, or cash value life insurance. A good agent will also urge you to obtain coverage that is essential to your well-being, even if it doesn't generate much commission. For example, if you haven't been told about the importance of umbrella liability insurance, you probably need a new agent.

Hopefully, you understand what it takes to be insured adequately. You can summarize your insurance status on the Insurance Coverage Checkup, and the Insurance Action Plan that follows can, with periodic reviews, keep you alert to insurance concerns that require your attention. You might be thinking that with all of the insurance you need you won't have any money left over. Don't worry. The next chapter is going to show you how to control your spending and get your debt under control so that you can not only afford to pay your insurance premiums, but also save money so that you can get rich—sensibly.

INSURANCE ACTION PLAN

	Current Status
Needs Action	Okay or Not Applicable

Needs Action	Okay or Not Applicable	
☐	☐	1. Review all your insurance coverage at least annually. Your insurance agent should orchestrate this review.
☐	☐	2. Prepare your own estimate of your life insurance needs. Don't rely on others to do it for you.
☐	☐	3. Be sure you or your agent get quotes from several companies prior to purchasing any life insurance.
☐	☐	4. If you need term insurance, be sure to check on any coverage that may be available through your employer and professional groups and associations.
☐	☐	5. If you have an estate that is likely to be near or in excess of $1,000,000, check with an estate planning attorney to assure that you have designated appropriate life insurance policy owners and beneficiaries.
☐	☐	6. Be sure that all family members, including parents and children who are out of the nest, have adequate and continuous health insurance.
☐	☐	7. Evaluate the sufficiency of the amount and the policy provisions of all disability insurance policies currently owned or provided by your employer.
☐	☐	8. If necessary, obtain additional disability coverage. Look for individually purchased policies with desirable features.
☐	☐	9. Take an inventory of your household possessions.

☐   ☐   10. Evaluate the adequacy of your homeowner's or renter's insurance and add to the coverage if you find any areas that are not fully insured.

☐   ☐   11. If you don't have professional liability for *all* of your professional endeavors, inquire as to your potential exposure. Take action to reduce this exposure if necessary.

☐   ☐   12. If you are considering any action to shield your assets from any potential medical lawsuits, seek legal counsel in advance.

☐   ☐   13. Obtain an extended personal liability (umbrella) policy if you haven't already.

☐   ☐   14. Consider increasing the amount of umbrella coverage if you now have only $1,000,000.

☐   ☐   15. Your insurance agent should be competent and responsive. If not, make a change.

3 | Physician, Heal Thy Spending and Borrowing Habits

HIGH INCOME CAN BE A MIXED BLESSING

How do you think people react when they meet a doctor or dentist? Do they envy your extensive training and skills, thinking, "How wonderful it must be to heal the afflicted"? Of course not. Rather, your occupation and social standing evoke different, albeit unarticulated feelings in people, such as, "I'd love to be making half of your income," or "I'll bet your tax bill *alone* is in the six figures." Unfortunately, it's more likely that the only thing in six figures is the doctor's annual carrying costs on a bunch of soured real estate deals.

In spite of popular lore, most health-care professionals are no different from their patients. They tend to spend and borrow more than they should, which, if not checked, impedes their progress toward financial security. In fact, a high and secure income may be a mixed blessing, since it can lead to excessive spending and inappropriate borrowing. Stories abound of once prosperous physicians and dentists who are struggling financially because of unwise investments that often were made on borrowed money.

- It should come as no surprise that highly compensated medical professionals can easily fall into the spending/borrowing trap.
- Years of costly education and poorly remunerated training

49

often leave newly minted doctors, dentists, and other health-care professionals saddled with substantial loans before they even begin their careers.

■ For those who choose to do so, the costs of establishing a practice often add to an already heavy loan burden.

■ Because of their job security and income prospects, doctors and dentists have long been wooed by lenders. The result in many instances has been too-easy credit.

■ The relatively high income enjoyed by many doctors and dentists makes it easy to establish a very comfortable, if not lavish life-style. All of the ingredients are there—income, easy credit, and visibility in the community. Everyone expects you to be one of the richest people in town, so you might as well live like you are. Sadly, as some people in your profession are beginning to find out, a life-style that consumes a continuing stream of high income cannot be maintained, if income is reduced.

■ Finally, many health-care professionals continue to sink considerable sums of money into real estate and other investments that require borrowing. This investment strategy used to be an effective means of reducing income taxes and, often, of creating wealth. However, the massive tax reforms of the 1980s virtually eliminated the tax-saving advantages of real estate investing, and the investment real estate market has hit the skids in most parts of the country. Nevertheless, many investors still have a Pavlovian response to real estate investments: If it's real estate, it has to be a good investment. Not true. Borrowing heavily to invest in real estate is, for most individual investors, a perilous course.

The above is not intended as an indictment of the entire health-care profession. Most members of the profession have their spending and borrowing under control. You are probably in reasonably good shape, but even so, there is always some room for improvement. So read on.

LEARNING TO CURB YOUR SPENDING APPETITE

The shortest routes to wealth are to marry it or inherit it. If neither applies to you, there is only one remaining alternative—to accumulate it yourself. I'll let you in on a secret—a surefire, can't-fail way to accumulate wealth: Spend less than you earn. I guess this must be a secret, because so few people do it. Why does this tautological concept elude so many of us? It is simply too easy to spend money. Our society rewards spending. People love to brag about their expensive automobiles and other possessions. How often do you hear people brag about the amount of money they save? Never, because if someone did, he or she would be branded as some sort of social misfit. Everyone would like to save, and everyone knows they need to save or to save more; but living beneath our means is tough, particularly for doctors, dentists, and other health-care professionals, many of whom have spent years living on a subsistence basis and then find themselves, almost overnight, with a high income.

How much should you save? At least 10 percent of your *gross* income, although 15 to 20 percent is, of course, better. While you may count any contributions that *you* make to your company's or your practice's retirement plans, you should also be saving some money outside the retirement plans. If you think I'm asking you to save too much, take a glance at Chapter 7, which covers retirement planning. It helps you estimate how much you will need to save (amass, really) by the time you retire. A high rate of savings may be particularly important for health-care professionals if, as many are predicting, people in the health-care business eventually go through a period of stagnant, or even declining earnings.

If you are having difficulty saving or would like to save more, you need to identify areas where you can reduce your spending and then find a way to save the money as painlessly as possible.

To spend is human; to save is divine.

EXPLORATORY SURGERY ON YOUR LIVING EXPENSES

Most people aren't too anxious to summarize how they spend their income, because they know they aren't going to like what they see. But you really should prepare a budget from time to time. A business can't operate effectively and efficiently without a budget, and your finances are really no different from a business's. The Personal Budget Planner included will enable you not only to summarize where you earn and spend your money now but also to plan for the future. This is what budgeting is all about. You know where you can cut down on expenses, and it is up to you and you alone to do so.

As you project your future expenses, be sure to take into account the many bills you pay on a less-than-monthly basis. It is these whopping bills that get so many of us in trouble. As luck would have it, most of them seem to come due at the same time, so just when we think we've got our expenses under control—*whammo!*—we owe our soul to some unfriendly insurance company. These are the kind of expenses that I'm talking about:

- Property taxes
- Homeowner's/renter's insurance
- Life insurance
- Professional liability insurance
- Other insurance
- Home improvements/maintenance
- Vacation
- Christmas/holidays
- Tuition
- Club membership dues
- Charitable contributions
- Estimated taxes
- IRA and Keogh plan contributions
- Furniture
- Seasonal fuel/electricity

If you never want to worry about these expenses again, add up how much they amount to annually, and each month deposit one-twelfth of that amount into a separate savings account. Of course, you must resist temptation and pay only those bills out of the account.

PERSONAL BUDGET PLANNER

This Personal Budget Planner can be used to record your past cash receipts and cash disbursements and/or to budget future receipts and disbursements. You may want to use the first column to record your past receipts and disbursements, the second column to list your budget over the next month, quarter, or year, and the third column to compare your actual future receipts and disbursements against your budget in the second column. If you budget over a period of less than one year, be sure to take into consideration those expenses that you pay less frequently than monthly, such as insurance, vacations, and tuition. You should be setting aside an amount each month that will eventually cover those large bills.

Indicate at the top of each column whether the amounts in that column are actual or estimated past figures or budgeted future figures. Also indicate the time period in each column—e.g., "July 1991" or "Year 1992."

Indicate if actual or budget: _____ _____ _____
Indicate the time period: _____ _____ _____

CASH RECEIPTS

1. Gross salary $_____ $_____ $_____
2. Interest _____ _____ _____
3. Dividends _____ _____ _____
4. Bonuses/profit sharing _____ _____ _____
5. Alimony/child support received _____ _____ _____
6. Distributions from partnerships _____ _____ _____
7. Income from outside businesses _____ _____ _____
8. Trust distributions _____ _____ _____
9. Pension _____ _____ _____
10. Social Security _____ _____ _____
11. Gifts _____ _____ _____
12. Proceeds from sale of investments _____ _____ _____
13. Other
   - _____ _____ _____
   - _____ _____ _____
   - _____ _____ _____
14. Total cash receipts $_____ $_____ $_____

CASH DISBURSEMENTS

1. Housing (rent/mortgage) $_____ $_____ $_____
2. Food _____ _____ _____
3. Household maintenance _____ _____ _____
4. Utilities and telephone _____ _____ _____
5. Clothing _____ _____ _____
6. Personal care _____ _____ _____
7. Medical and dental care _____ _____ _____
8. Automobile/transportation _____ _____ _____
9. Child care expenses _____ _____ _____
10. Entertainment _____ _____ _____
11. Vacation(s) _____ _____ _____

12. Gifts   _____ _____ _____
13. Contributions   _____ _____ _____
14. Insurance   _____ _____ _____
15. Miscellaneous out-of-pocket
    expenses   _____ _____ _____
16. Furniture   _____ _____ _____
17. Home improvements   _____ _____ _____
18. Real estate taxes   _____ _____ _____
19. Loan payments   _____ _____ _____
20. Credit card payments   _____ _____ _____
21. Alimony/child support
    payments   _____ _____ _____
22. Tuition/educational expenses _____ _____ _____
23. Business and professional
    expenses   _____ _____ _____
24. Savings/investments   _____ _____ _____
25. Income and Social Security
    taxes   _____ _____ _____
26. Other
    ■_____   _____ _____ _____
    ■_____   _____ _____ _____
    ■_____   _____ _____ _____
27. Total cash disbursements $_____ $_____ $_____

EXCESS (SHORTFALL) OF
CASH RECEIPTS OVER
CASH DISBURSEMENTS $_____ $_____ $_____

BETTER LIVING THROUGH ELECTRONICS

The easiest way to save money is never to see it. Bankers and credit union managers have told me time and again that the customers who really amass a lot of money over the years do it through payroll deduction or by some other means of having their money taken from them regularly—*electronically.* It doesn't have to be taken out of your paycheck. Most financial institutions (including mutual fund companies) are more than happy to help you not to see your money, and all you have to do is authorize them to withdraw a certain amount of money from your checking account each week or each month and place it in some investment account. However you choose to save, be sure to save regularly. By the way, the next time your salary increases, increase the amount of savings that you have deducted from your paycheck or bank account.

Say no to spending. Get high on saving.

DEBT—A DOUBLE-EDGED SCALPEL

Interest on debt used to save higher income people a lot on their taxes. But times have changed. Consumer indebtedness, which is just about all kinds of debt except home mortgages and investment loans, is no longer tax deductible. Even tax-deductible debt doesn't save much in taxes anymore, since tax rates are now so much lower than they used to be. Interest amounting to $10,000 used to save a high-income taxpayer $5,000 in federal income taxes. It currently saves far less than that, if it is deductible at all. Any way you incise it, debt is less attractive than it used to be, but judging by the ever-increasing level of credit-card indebtedness, that hasn't deterred many people from borrowing.

Debt can be very beneficial, or it can be detrimental. Just as you can distinguish between essential spending and frivolous spending, you know that there are good reasons to borrow and bad reasons to borrow. If you list your current loans and what they were used to purchase, you will be able to make that distinction easily.

THE KEYS TO GOOD DEBT MANAGEMENT

The best way to manage personal debt is to borrow only for appropriate reasons and to pay off the loans within a reasonable period of time. Good debt finances something worthwhile that will benefit you well into the future. Bad debt usually finances something that you use up almost immediately or that you never receive any real benefit from (borrowing to consolidate loans, for example). Thus, a home mortgage is good debt, and credit card indebtedness is almost always bad debt. Borrowing to invest in real estate can be either good or bad, depending upon how the investment fares. Unfortunately, some investors, and medical professionals are all too well represented among them, buy into real estate projects that are doomed from the outset.

All loans should be paid off as soon as possible—ideally, long before the asset you purchased with the loan stops benefiting you. Car loans are a special case, since they involve borrowing to buy a depreciating asset. Therefore, a car should be financed over no more than two or three years, although the average car loan is now almost five years. If you borrow for much more than two years, you will be incurring repair bills while still making loan payments on your metal and plastic master. This is hardly an appealing situation. If you can't afford to finance a car over less than three years, you can't afford that car. It's hard to believe, but younger people typically spend more to own and maintain a car then they do on housing. No wonder they can't seem to save up enough to make a down payment on a home.

HOME SWEET HOME MORTGAGE

You may benefit handsomely by accelerating the repayment of your home mortgage. As a general rule of thumb, unless you can earn a return on an investment that is greater than the interest rate on your mortgage, you are better off making an additional payment against your mortgage. Don't spend every last dime trying to reduce your mortgage, however. You should always keep sufficient resources on hand to tide you over in case of an emergency. Aside from that, however, accelerating the repayment of the mortgage can save a great deal of money.

> *Example:* Helen Homestead, an RN, recently took out a $100,000, thirty-year fixed mortgage at 10 percent interest. Her monthly mortgage payment is $878. If she pays another $197 per month against the mortgage, she will pay off the loan in fifteen years, rather than thirty years, and save around $90,000 on the total after-tax cost of the mortgage.

You should try, if possible, to pay off your mortgage by the time you retire, because it will greatly reduce the amount of income you will need to retire comfortably.

Mortgage refinancing is another matter that you may want to address if you currently have a high interest fixed-rate mortgage, or if you are uncomfortable with your adjustable-rate mortgage. While some rules of thumb may help you assess whether the time is right to consider refinancing, you will have to put pencil to paper to decide. You must weigh the costs of refinancing against the longer term interest savings. But if you expect to stay in the house for the next several years, and prevailing interest rates are one or two percent lower than your current mort-

> Some doctors and dentists have been so enamored of real estate investing that their finances are now in critical condition.

gage rate, you may benefit from refinancing, particularly if current fixed mortgage rates are in the single digits.

HELs BELLS

Hardly a day goes by without some lender ringing the bells in celebration of home equity loans—and with good reason. HELs are one of the best loan arrangements ever invented—for the lenders, anyway. What they're pushing is a variable rate secured loan. A lender can't ask for much more than that. What you're getting is a convenient, and perhaps tempting source of money, the interest on which, depending upon your circumstances, is probably tax deductible. For good managers of family credit, home equity loans may be the preferable borrowing source. For the easily tempted they can be downright dangerous.

To be useful, home equity credit lines must be managed like any other loan—by paying off the outstanding balance over an appropriate period of time. If you draw on your credit line to pay income taxes or to take a vacation (either of which should have been anticipated and otherwise provided for), the loan balance should be paid off quickly—within a few months at most. If you use the credit line to buy a car, pay it off over two or three years, just like you should an automobile loan. There are only a couple of uses of home equity loan money—or any loan money, for that matter—that would justify a long repayment period. First is if you make *substantive* improvements to your home in lieu of moving. Substantive does not mean a swimming pool or bocce court, but something that adds significant value to your home, like adding another bedroom or remodeling your kitchen. A long repayment term may also be justified if you use the money to pay college tuition for your children. If you do hock the home for this very worthwhile purpose, you should do so only after all other possible scholarship, grant, and loan sources have been exhausted.

PLANNING TO MEET LIFE'S MAJOR EXPENSES

STARTING A PRACTICE

According to a Department of Commerce survey, there were 235,000 doctor's offices in the United States, of which 116,000 were individual practices, 9,000 were partnerships, and the remainder were professional corporations. While an increasing number of recent medical and dental school graduates are opting for salaried positions with regular hours, better family life, and less debt, many are still interested in eventually opening their own individual practices. If you are contemplating this career path, be forewarned of the high cost of opening an office or purchasing an existing practice, which may add to an already high student-loan burden. Well in advance of starting or acquiring a practice, you should consult with a lawyer and an accountant who are experienced in advising doctors on these matters. They will be able to help you with a number of important matters, including the best way to organize the practice, i.e., proprietorship, partnership, or professional corporation, and if you are acquiring an existing practice, they can advise you as to an appropriate price to pay. They will also be able to help you negotiate the purchase.

Unless you are awash with cash, you will also have to finance the newly acquired or started practice. You must not, however, saddle yourself with too much debt. You will be required to prepare projections of estimated revenues and expenses from the practice to justify the loan, but this is an essential exercise for your own planning purposes anyway. The following table breaks down the cost of operating a typical medical or dental office. It may help you plan for the purchase of a practice, or to compare your figures if you already own a practice.

Don't let the excitement of putting out your shingle cloud your judgment. Also, remember that income prospects in the medical and dental professions may not be as rosy as they have been. But if you use good judgment to start the practice and you retain and use experienced counsel, you will be well on your way to professional as well as financial independence.

BUYING A FIRST HOME

One of the best things you can do to achieve financial independence is to buy a home, whether it's a house, condominium,

COST BREAKDOWN OF A MEDICAL OR DENTAL OFFICE

	Doctors' Offices	Dentists' Offices
Operating costs	8.5%	15.7%
Officer's compensation*	40.2	29.1
Pensions and benefits	10.4	6.8
Rent	4.0	4.8
Repairs	0.4	0.5
Depreciation & amortization	2.3	2.9
Interest	0.5	0.7
Bad debts	0.1	—
Advertising	0.1	0.6
State, local taxes	2.6	3.4
Other expenses	30.1	33.2
Net profit before tax	0.8	2.3

*Includes doctor's or dentist's salary.

Source: *1983–1984 Almanac of Business and Industrial Financial Ratios* by Leo Troy.

cooperative, duplex, triplex, or town house. For most people, the advantages of owning far outweigh the disadvantages. True, interest rates may be high and housing prices flat or declining. Some people wait around for ideal conditions—low interest rates and housing prices that are low but poised to go through the stratosphere. These people usually become permanent renters, because conditions will never be so ideal. Don't worry too much about current conditions. Concentrate instead on saving for the down payment, becoming familiar with the local real estate market, and putting your overall finances in good order so you can qualify for a mortgage. Lenders are getting stricter, so don't be surprised if they make you jump through hoops prior to granting the mortgage. Fortunately, your occupation will be a big plus. Finally, don't set your sights too high on a first home. Most first-time home buyers start out in a home and neighborhood that aren't quite as nice as the ones they grew up in. Eventually you'll be able to trade up, but for now the important thing is to get into

There has to be divine guidance in life because spenders tend to marry savers.

that first home. You'll probably be temporarily impoverished by the home purchase, but that's good practice for future life events that may also impoverish you, like educating the kids.

EDUCATING YOUR CHILDREN

Have you educated yourself on education costs? Educating the children is, for many parents, one of their biggest financial challenges. Careful planning is essential. The only thing that can be said for certain about future college costs is that they will continue to outpace inflation. You will probably not qualify for any financial aid. Right now, a family with total assets of $80,000, including the equity in their home and with total income of $60,000, would probably *not* qualify for any financial aid for a child in college. Even if you enjoy a comfortable income, you may still have difficulty meeting college tuition bills. Fortunately, colleges and lending institutions have invented innovative ways to help beleaguered families meet these costs. Many colleges offer tuition prepayment plans that allow you to pay for all four years of college at the first year's rate. Some colleges even lend parents the funds to do this with extended repayment schedules of up to fifteen years. The following College Education Funding Forecaster work sheet can help you project how much you will need to save to meet college education costs.

Loan sources are more abundant than outright assistance, but overreliance on loans can end up saddling you or your child with too much debt. If you take the time to evaluate loan sources carefully, you will often be rewarded by uncovering loans with lower interest rates and more flexible repayment schedules.

One last thing. Don't rely on what your friends say about college financial aid matters. Conditions change so rapidly that the tips they give are probably out of date. Good information is available from local high schools and colleges and from numerous publications.

Below is a spending and borrowing action plan to help you keep your expenses under control. Now that you've got a clear picture of your current financial situation and a solid foundation to work from, it's time to move on to that appealing and elusive stage, accumulating wealth.

COLLEGE EDUCATION FUNDING FORECASTER WORK SHEET

This work sheet can help you estimate how much you will need to save each year in order to fund future college expenses. The college education *cost* forecaster projects average college education costs for a four-year public or private school education. The college education *savings* estimator calculates how much you will have to save to meet those costs.

College Education Cost Forecaster

The following table (compiled by the College Board) projects current average four-year education costs, assuming a 6 percent annual increase in costs. These figures can be used as a guide in estimating the costs of college for your child or children.

Year Entering	Public School	Private School	Selective Private School
1991	$24,405	$ 62,104	$ 87,690
1992	25,870	65,831	92,951
1993	27,422	69,780	98,528
1994	29,067	73,967	104,440
1995	30,811	78,405	110,706
1996	32,660	83,110	117,348
1997	34,620	88,096	124,389
1998	36,697	93,382	131,853
1999	38,899	98,985	139,764
2000	41,232	104,923	148,150
2001	43,706	111,219	157,039
2002	46,329	117,893	166,461
2003	49,109	124,966	176,449
2004	52,055	132,464	187,036
2005	55,178	140,412	198,258
2006	58,489	148,837	210,153
2007	61,998	157,767	222,762
2008	65,718	167,233	236,127
2009	69,661	177,267	250,295
2010	73,841	187,903	265,313

College Education Savings Estimator

Name of Child				Total
1. Total estimated college costs (from above)	$	$	$	$
2. Amount of savings currently available for college[1]	$	$	$	
3. Multiplied by appreciation factor (from table below)[2]	x	x	x	
4. Equals estimated amount of current savings available at college age (Line 2 times Line 3)	$	$	$	
5. Estimated amount of costs remaining to be funded (Line 1 minus Line 4)	$	$	$	
6. Adjustments[3]	$	$	$	
7. Equals amount that you wish to accumulate by college age (Line 5 plus/ minus Line 6)	$	$	$	$
8. Multiplied by accumulation factor from table below[4]	x	x	x	

9. Equals the
   amount to be
   saved each year
   to meet future
   college costs[5] $_____ $_____ $_____ $_____

APPRECIATION   FACTOR   TABLE   FOR   LINE   3

Year Child Enters College	Factor	Year Child Enters College	Factor
1991	1.07	2001	2.11
1992	1.15	2002	2.25
1993	1.23	2003	2.41
1994	1.31	2004	2.58
1995	1.40	2005	2.76
1996	1.50	2006	2.94
1997	1.60	2007	3.15
1998	1.72	2008	3.37
1999	1.84	2009	3.61
2000	1.97	2010	3.87

ACCUMULATION   FACTOR   TABLE   FOR   LINE   8

Year Child Enters College	Factor	Year Child Enters College	Factor
1991	.483	2001	.056
1992	.311	2002	.050
1993	.225	2003	.044
1994	.174	2004	.040
1995	.140	2005	.036
1996	.116	2006	.032
1997	.097	2007	.027
1998	.083	2008	.027
1999	.072	2009	.024
2000	.063	2010	.022

Notes:
    1. Indicate on Line 2 any savings you now have that are earmarked to pay education costs. Many parents with more than one child simply divide these savings equally among the children unless the savings or investment accounts are in a specified child's name.
    2. The appreciation factor on Line 3 is provided in the Appreciation Factor table. It recognizes the future increase in value of the savings or investments that you presently have earmarked for college costs. The factor assumes a 7 percent annual increase in value.
    3. Many parents will want to make adjustments in Line 6 to the estimated amount of

college costs to be funded. Reductions might be appropriate in situations where financial aid can reasonably be anticipated or where the child will be expected to contribute to college costs through summer or school-year income. Additions to the estimated costs to be funded will be appropriate if, for example, the parent expects the child to go to a college that is more expensive than average. Selective private colleges, in particular, may be considerably more expensive than the averages provided on this work sheet.

4. The accumulation factor to be entered on Line 8 is provided in the Accumulation Factor table. Multiplying this factor by the amount of money that you wish to accumulate by college age will show the amount of money that you would need to save each year to accumulate the necessary funds. An annual return of 7 percent is assumed.

5. Parents are often dismayed by the amount of money that they would have to save each year to meet future college costs (Line 9). Don't be discouraged, however. The important thing to do is to begin a regular savings program even if it's only a portion of the amount indicated. Remember also that the annual amount to be saved assumes *level* payment. Even if you can afford to save only a portion of the amount indicated on Line 9, you will still be able to accumulate a nest egg that will go a long way toward easing the financial burden of your children's education. It is often more realistic for parents to gradually increase the amount of money they set aside each year.

SPENDING AND BORROWING ACTION PLAN

Current Status

Needs Action	Okay or Not Applicable	
☐	☐	1. Save at least 10 percent of your gross income.
☐	☐	2. Maintain a life-style that your income can support comfortably.
☐	☐	3. Prepare a budget from time to time to summarize your income and expenditures.
☐	☐	4. If you have trouble paying large bills, set up a separate savings account for that purpose.
☐	☐	5. Create an emergency savings fund equal to about three months' expenses.
☐	☐	6. Borrow only for worthwhile purposes.
☐	☐	7. If you can afford it, make additional payments on your home mortgage from time to time.

☐ ☐ 8. If and when conditions warrant, consider refinancing your home in the current interest rate environment.

☐ ☐ 9. If you are contemplating starting your own practice or purchasing a practice, consult with both a lawyer and an accountant.

☐ ☐ 10. If applicable, take action now to provide for your children's education.

Comments:_____
_____
_____
_____
_____
_____

Spending and Borrowing "To Do" List:_____
_____
_____
_____
_____
_____

II

ACCUMULATING WEALTH

4 | A Prescription for Investment Success

Investing wisely is arguably the most important thing you will do to achieve financial security. It's just about as easy to make good investments as it is to make dumb investments. Most people don't make dumb investments on their own, rather, someone encourages them. Therefore, in this chapter and the one that follows we will help you become a better investor—one who can make sensible investment decisions independent of some biased outsider's suggestions. These chapters emphasize investing in each of the three major investment categories—stock investments, interest-earning investments, and real estate investments. Nevertheless, you should not lose sight of other important "investments" that directly or indirectly will contribute to your ultimate financial success, including your career, your pension plans, your home, good health, and a stable personal life.

As the following diagram illustrates, investing is really the focal point of the personal financial planning process.

As important as investing is, most people don't do a very good job at it. What's the secret to successful investing? First, you must decide what you want to accomplish with your investments. Generally, you will ultimately want to use them to provide retirement income, although you may be interrupted along the way to meet such important needs as buying a first home and educating the children. As corny as it sounds, if you don't have some clearly identified idea of what you're going to do with the money, you're not going to be able to organize your investments

FIGURE 1

Investing Is the Focal Point of the Personal Financial Planning Process

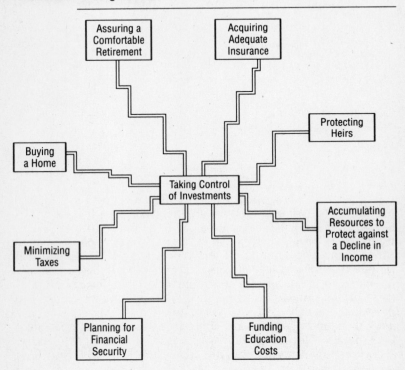

to meet those targets. Once you have set realistic objectives, you can then go about making investments that will help you achieve them. The right kind of investments are undoubtedly ones that you are already pretty familiar with. They are not new types of investments, neither are they the kinds of investments that you have to buy and sell all the time. In a word, they're "old-fashioned." Finally, successful investors, whether they do it themselves or use investment advisers, won't let anyone persuade them to alter their objectives or their investments significantly.

Example: A good friend of mine who is a very successful stockbroker as well as radio talk show host related the following true story to me: "A few years ago a recently retired man came into my office to ask for some investment advice. He said that he was very embarrassed about his situation and had avoided speaking with an investment adviser about it for several years. About twenty-five years earlier he had inherited $40,000 worth of stock from his father. He told me that at that time he didn't know anything about investments, although he recognized the names of all the companies whose shares he had inherited. So he put the stock certificates in his safe-deposit box, where they sat for twenty-five years. He then went on to say that he had been receiving dividend income all along, and he noted that it had increased considerably over the years. I told him to retrieve the certificates from the safe-deposit box so we could figure out what they were worth. Well, as you might suspect, his stock was now worth over $500,000. I shudder to think what would have happened if he had asked someone to manage these investments actively over the past twenty-five years rather than having put them in the safe-deposit box." The moral of this story: Sometimes the best thing to do is nothing.

A number of issues make investment planning for doctors and dentists unique:

■ Medical professionals are likely to be highly compensated, but no matter how successful their practices are, they do not build up value the way other businesses do. Most doctors and dentists have built their economic life around their practices, which usually have a low market value and restricted transferability. Since this limits their estate planning and retirement options severely, health-care professionals must rely more heavily on accumulating sufficient personal investments to provide adequately for retirement and their heirs. In addition, growing concerns that their income may trend downward should affect doctors' and dentists' investment decisions.

■ Because of their extensive training, most medical professionals begin their careers relatively late, and many begin heavily in debt. A shorter working life means they have to accumulate more during their working years. In addition, many doctors and dentists, especially those in private practice, either fund their own pension plans or do not participate in pension plans.

■ Doctors and dentists tend to fall into a common pattern with regard to their own investment strategies as well. They typically are too busy to manage their investments appropriately, and consequently may rely too heavily on their investment advisers. High incomes lead many of them to be overly concerned with the tax ramifications of their investments. Some of them are fond of devising elaborate schemes for depriving Uncle Sam of his money, heedless of how much they deprive themselves. They tend not to coordinate their investment planning with their estate planning. Finally, remarkably few health-care professionals exploit their own unique abilities to identify and invest in, for example, promising medical and pharmaceutical stocks. Some cynics have observed that doctors and dentists have to earn a lot of money because they end up losing most of it through lousy investments.

Why do so many medical professionals have difficulty accumulating and managing their investments? While their occupational status is unique, I'm not so sure that their problems are much different from those of the general populace—it's just that the size of their mistakes is often much larger.

In the course of my work with physicians and dentists over the years, I have found that many—though certainly not all—tend to fall into one or more of the following investment traps:

- They abdicate (rather than delegate) responsibility for investment selection and management to others.
- They are too trusting of investment salespeople.
- They do not save enough in relation to their income, particularly when they are younger and middle-aged.
- They have unrealistic expectations of the appropriate return on their investments and become impatient when their advisers fall short of these expectations.
- They tend to invest in extremes. Some take far too much risk while others are overly conservative.
- They fail to take a long-term view of investing. Instead they react to fads and the opinions of the uninformed.

SETTING OBJECTIVES

Everyone's primary financial planning goal is financial security. Financial security means that your investments (combined with Social Security and pension benefits) will provide you and your dependents with an adequate income for the rest of your life. In essence, financial security means you can afford to retire. Some people achieve financial security sooner than others. Some people never achieve it. Most of us want to be financially secure no later than retirement age.

It is very difficult for the medical professional to create wealth by building up his or her practice. The goodwill created by the practice does not command a significant price from the eventual buyer of the practice, if any. Therefore, you must be particularly careful to assure that sufficient current income is set aside to provide for any unforeseen contingencies as well as an adequate retirement.

Accumulating sufficient personal capital is the single most important component of financial security. This is particularly true for medical professionals, since most are responsible for funding their own retirement income needs. If this describes your situation, the contents of this chapter apply every bit as much to your pension plan investments as they do to investments outside the pension plan. Also, remember that financial security requires that all areas of financial planning—including insurance, tax planning, and estate planning—be attended to. For example, you may eventually accumulate a whopping estate, but if you are not properly and completely insured, you are not financially secure. These topics are discussed elsewhere in this book.

One of the most important elements of long-term investment success is *consistency*. Far too many medical professionals blindly throw their money away, following "hot" market tips and their commissioned purveyor's breathless recommendations about financial products with seductive sales raps but dubious merit, such items as "unbundled stock units," "payment in kind preferred stock," or "equity index participations." Whether you are just embarking on a saving-and-investing program or are in midvoyage, you need to establish and periodically review your investment objectives. These need to be clearly articulated in each of the following areas:

1. The amount or percentage of earnings to be set aside periodically for investment purposes. If you aren't yet sure how much you will need to save, you can get a better idea in Chapter 7, where you will figure out how much you need to save in order to be able to retire comfortably.

2. A reasonable target long-term rate of return on investments. Permit me to give you a target. You should strive to earn a return on your investments that exceeds inflation by at least 3 percent after taxes. This is easier said than done, however. I would suggest that for planning purposes you assume a 4 to 5 percent long-term inflation rate. As the example below indicates, if your combined federal and state tax rate is 33 percent, you would have to earn a 12-percent return on a taxable interest-earning investment—such as a CD—in order to beat inflation by 3 percent after taxes. It'll be less confusing after the example.

FIGURE 2

Comparison of Interest-Earning Investments That Pay 10% Interest and 12% Interest.

	Rate of Return	
	10%	12%
Pretax income on a $10,000 investment	$1,000	$1,200
Federal income tax (28%)	(280)	(336)
State income tax (5%)	(50)	(60)
Total tax	(330)	(396)
After-tax income	$ 670	$ 804
After-tax return on the $10,000 investment	6.7%	8.0%

Note:
If the inflation rate is 5 percent, the investment that pays 10 percent interest beats inflation by only 1.7 percent, while the 12 percent return investment (if one can be found) beats inflation by 3 percent.

Most investors don't realize the impact of taxes. When CD rates reach nine or ten percent, many investors think they have died and gone to heaven. Yet, on an after-tax basis, they are staying just ahead of inflation. On the other hand, these rates are *very* attractive for retirement-oriented accounts, since retirement funds are not taxed until they are withdrawn at retirement. So an 8.5 percent CD is growing at 8.5 percent per year—well ahead of inflation. This is one of many good reasons why you need to maximize your retirement account contributions and take advantage of other sensible tax-deferred investments that are discussed in Chapter 6.

3. The third objective involves the allocation of your investments among the three major investment categories, which are stocks, interest-earning securities, and real estate, so that you will be able to achieve the desired rate of return without subjecting your investments to undue risk. These matters are discussed in the next chapter.

MAXIMIZING YOUR INVESTMENT SAVVY WITH A MINIMUM TIME INVESTMENT

Before you can take control of your own finances, you must have at least some understanding of the various types of investments available. The more understanding you gain, the better; but the demands of a medical career typically preclude you from becoming an investment expert or staying up-to-date with the ever-changing investment markets. However, those who have too little knowledge of or interest in investments are more often than not going to suffer, either at the hands of opportunistic "advisers" or by just plain overlooking or avoiding an appropriate investment.

> *Example:* One of my doctor clients, who came to me as he was nearing retirement, had the entirety of his wealth invested in money market accounts and rural raw land. He thought he was investing safely and conservatively, but actually he was losing purchasing power because his investments were barely keeping up with inflation. With no stocks, no bonds, and no income-producing real estate, he hadn't balanced his portfolio properly. I'm sure he could have done worse with his investments, but he also could have done much better. He hadn't taken the time to learn about the other investment categories, and he didn't trust anyone else to advise him in these matters.

The following table will help you understand the kinds of commonly used—and usually sensible—investments that you might include in your portfolio. Some may be suitable for you, others not. It depends upon your objectives. The table is organized according to the three major investment categories: stock, interest-earning, and real estate. Within each category, the investment securities are organized according to the way in which you purchase and own them, either directly by buying the securities yourself, or indirectly through mutual funds; or in the case of real estate, through limited partnerships. The fine points of investing are discussed in the next chapter.

> I just saw my doctor walk into her office with *The Wall Street Journal* tucked under her arm. I had an uneasy feeling in my stomach. But I guess things could be worse, like seeing my stockbroker reading *Practical Gastroenterology*.

INVESTMENT BILL OF FARE

COMMON STOCK INVESTMENTS

Directly owned (owning shares of stock of individual companies):

INCOME STOCKS pay a high dividend and are usually in fairly stable industries, like public utilities. Popular with retirees and bank trust departments.

GROWTH STOCKS are bought for capital appreciation, because they pay little or no dividend. Can be as volatile as all get out.

BLUE CHIP STOCKS are sometimes referred to as "blue gyp" stocks. High quality, steadily increasing dividend. A lot of wealthy families got that way by investing solely in blue chips, which should tell you something.

CYCLICAL STOCKS are shares of companies whose earnings tend to fluctuate with their business cycles, such as steel and housing. Cyclicals don't always behave like the pundits say they should; otherwise, no one would own their shares when the business cycle turns down.

SPECULATIVE STOCKS are brilliant investments if they go up. Otherwise, it's gambling, but certainly a better form of gambling than playing the lottery, which is nothing more than a tax on the naive. Like any form of gambling, don't bet heavily on speculative issues.

Indirectly owned (owning shares of stock mutual funds, which in turn own shares of the stock of many corporations):

AGGRESSIVE GROWTH FUNDS, also known as maximum capital gains funds, seek the greatest possible gain, and often invest in speculative stocks. They do great in bull markets and terribly in bear markets. Long-term holders of these funds have been amply rewarded in the past.

GROWTH AND INCOME FUNDS aim for a reasonable return by combining growth stocks with higher quality dividend-paying stocks. More conservative than aggressive growth funds, and still show solid returns.

BALANCED FUNDS usually invest about half their assets or more in stocks and the balance in bonds or other debt instruments. Good way to get an instantly diversified stock and bond portfolio, for an investment of $1,000 or less. My favorite investment.

INTERNATIONAL FUNDS are the only efficient way to invest in foreign stocks, and foreign stocks belong in every well-diversified portfolio.

GOLD FUNDS invest in, you guessed it, gold, or more likely, the shares of gold-mining companies. People hold gold as a hedge against inflation. Short of buying and storing the bullion (ingots are very impressive paperweights), this is the best way to play the gold market.

INTEREST-EARNING INVESTMENTS

Directly owned (owning the securities of individual bond or certificate issuers):

TREASURY SECURITIES are the means by which the U.S. government borrows money—and as you know, they're pretty good at borrowing money. Treasury bills, notes, and bonds are issued regularly by the Fed and are a popular investment, particularly for people who are averse to risk and are averse to paying state income taxes.

MORTGAGE-BACKED SECURITIES have names that sound like characters on *Hee Haw*, like Ginnie Mae, Fannie Mae, and Freddie Mac. These investments represent interests in pools of mortgages. Their relatively high yields have been attracting a lot of investor interest, but high investment minimums, typically $25,000, keep out the riffraff.

MUNICIPAL BONDS don't appeal to people who enjoy paying federal income taxes, which means they're very popular. If you purchase bonds of issuing authorities in your own state (or bonds of Puerto Rico), you escape state income taxes and, perhaps, local income taxes.

CORPORATE BONDS, of course, represent debt obligations of corporations and vary significantly in quality from triple-A rated all the way down to junk bonds. Purchasers of junk bonds (issuers prefer to call them "high yield" bonds) know well the perils of blindly chasing the highest yielding corporate bond issues.

CERTIFICATES OF DEPOSIT are interest-bearing deposits with banks, with a specified maturity that typically ranges from thirty days to five or more years. Federally insured CDs are a major form of investment for many people. They shouldn't be, because better yields are usually available through other interest-earning investments.

Indirectly owned (owning shares of fixed-income mutual funds or money market funds, which in turn own interest-earning debt obligations of many issuers):

GOVERNMENT SECURITIES FUNDS invest in Treasury securities and/or mortgage-backed securities. Low investment minimums on these funds provide investors of all means with access to the government securities markets.

MUNICIPAL BOND FUNDS are available aplenty, including single-state funds that provide double tax exemption to residents of a particular state. Similar to all mutual funds that invest in long-term debt obligations, muni funds can decline in value if prevailing interest rates rise.

CORPORATE BOND FUNDS pay higher interest than municipal funds, but what you have left over after paying income taxes on the interest paid out by the corporate bond fund is what matters. Similar to municipal bond funds, each corporate bond fund states in its prospectus the quality of the bonds it will buy for its portfolio. Therefore, investors can select funds that invest in anywhere from the highest to the lowest quality bonds.

MONEY MARKET FUNDS invest in short-term, usually very safe and stable, securities, including commercial paper (short-term IOUs of large U.S. corporations), Treasury bills, and large bank CDs. Money funds are a very convenient place to stash your money and allow it to earn at least some interest while stashed.

REAL ESTATE INVESTMENTS

Directly owned (owning and managing a real estate investment):

INCOME-PRODUCING REAL ESTATE can range from a rented condominium unit to an apartment building to commercial properties. These are attractive investments with possible tax benefits, although many medical professionals lack the time or inclination to manage income-producing real estate.

UNDEVELOPED LAND ties up a lot of money for a long time. Land in particularly desirable areas is very expensive, but with some luck, it will appreciate smartly.

Indirectly owned (purchasing an interest in a real estate limited partnership):

REAL ESTATE LIMITED PARTNERSHIPS, once the darling of the tax-shelter devotees, have fallen on hard times. The loss of tax benefits, combined with overbuilding in many locales, has left many limited partnership investors disillusioned—and a lot poorer. Attractive deals are still possible, but buyer beware!

Once you become familiar with the different types of investments, you need to understand the concept of a balanced portfolio and decide how best to allocate your own resources among the three major categories of investment assets: stock investments, interest-earning investments, and real estate investments. Don't confuse this with the notion of "market timing" that is currently in vogue. Market timing means that someone purports to be able to divine the optimum proportion of assets invested in the various investment categories at any point in time. Of course, these proportions change faster than Bolivia's government. Short-term market timing just doesn't work well. On the other hand, the concept of asset allocation is terribly important in planning your "permanent portfolio structure." In short, you need to establish some general parameters to guide your portfolio mix, for example, "My portfolio will consist roughly of 40 percent stocks, 30 percent bonds, and 30 percent real estate." More on this in the next chapter.

Medical professionals usually lack the time and often lack the knowledge to monitor their investments to their satisfaction. If this is your situation, it is particularly important for you to select your investment advisers carefully, and review their performance regularly as well. Finally, developing a general knowledge of investment techniques and current market conditions will make you a much more effective client.

SOME GENERAL INVESTMENT RULES OF THUMB

INVEST WITH A LONG-TERM VIEW. Although your broker may not want me to say this, the buy-and-hold strategy of investing usually produces much better results (for the investor) than an actively traded portfolio. Studies have shown that over most holding periods of ten years or longer, investors in stocks have enjoyed returns well in excess of inflation; shorter holding periods generally produce much lower returns. Also, if you take a long-term perspective, you will certainly fret less over short-term market vacillations.

BUY QUALITY. Quality investments offer a good measure of protection, particularly in times of market volatility and investment uncertainty. Stocks and bonds of well-established companies, or well-located real estate investments, have greater staying power when market conditions deteriorate. Buy only those mutual funds that have produced above-average performance over the past five to ten years.

DON'T BORROW TO INVEST IN ANYTHING EXCEPT REAL ESTATE. The investors who were really hurt by the adverse bond and stock market conditions of 1987 were generally those who borrowed on margin to increase their investments. The only way for them to cover their margin calls was to sell their holdings at an inopportune time. While borrowing for real estate can be an effective means of increasing investment returns, heavily margined stock and bond investors expose themselves to considerable risk.

The only three reasons why your stockbroker would want you to sell a stock:
1. It has fallen in value and doesn't look as good as it once did. There are better opportunities in other stocks.
2. It's at the same price as when you bought it; it just isn't moving. There are better opportunities in other stocks.
3. It has risen in value. Let's lock in your profits now. There are better opportunities in other stocks. (This occurrence is exceedingly rare but has been known to happen.)

AVOID HIGH-RISK INVESTMENTS. While you may think they offer you a one-way ticket to nirvana, commodities, futures, coins, and stock options are, for the most part, suckers' games. If you want to make high-risk investments, feel free so long as you use only a small portion of your portfolio. Just be prepared to lose the money, because more often than not, lose it you will.

AVOID NEW INVESTMENTS. Don't buy anything new, such as a new stock issue (you probably aren't important enough to your broker to be offered an issue that will rise in value), a new closed-end fund (they almost always go down in value), a new piece of real estate (it doesn't have a rent history), or a new and improved type of security. Don't be a guinea pig.

SHOP AROUND FOR THE BEST INTEREST RATES ON INTEREST-EARNING INVESTMENTS. Take advantage of competition in the marketplace by shopping for the best rates. For example, ask your broker to quote a "brokered CD" rate. CDs that are sold through brokers often pay higher interest than you can fetch at your local bank. The same goes for money market funds. Money market mutual funds usually offer much higher yields than bank money market deposit accounts.

VARY THE MATURITIES ON INTEREST-EARNING INVESTMENTS. You should avoid concentrating the maturities of your interest-

Ten percent "sure" is better than 25 percent "maybe."

earning investments. For example, rather than buying a single two-year CD, consider splitting it up among a one-year, two-year, and five-year CD. By staggering (also known as "laddering") maturities, you will avoid being stuck with, say, a lot of long-term bonds during a period of rising interest rates. If you were, the value of your bonds would drop, and therefore you would be stuck with low-interest-rate investments. Another thing you can do with interest-earning investments is to time their maturities to coincide with years when you will need the cash—when the children are in college, or during your retirement years. If you invest in bond mutual funds, you can still stagger maturities by dividing up your fund investments among short-term, intermediate-term, and longer-term bond funds.

BUY NO-LOAD MUTUAL FUNDS. You will do yourself a favor by spending a little time researching mutual funds, and selecting no-load mutual funds with low annual expenses. Rest assured that if you buy a fund through a broker, even if it's a "no load," the broker is getting paid, and it's coming out of your investment. Whatever your particular investment need, there's a true no-load fund that will meet it. Some fund families, including Dreyfus, Fidelity, T. Rowe Price, Twentieth Century, and Vanguard, provide a multitude of excellent no-load or low-load funds that are operated very efficiently.

Investing is the focal point of successful personal financial planning. Yet many medical professionals don't do a very good job with their investments. Up to this point, we have laid the groundwork for a more detailed review of how you can build an investment portfolio that will help you on your way to achieving financial security. This is the subject of the next chapter. But first, you should review the following table, which summarizes my personal and admittedly biased assessment of the suitability of various types of investments.

If someone who is trying to sell you an investment can't explain it to your satisfaction in one sentence, don't buy it.

TABLE 4

Pond's Assessment of Investment Suitability

TYPE OF INVESTMENT	ASSESSMENT
Equity Investments:	
Common stock	Has been, is, and will continue to be good long-term inflation hedge. Buy and hold.
Preferred stock	Not very exciting unless you want the dividend income.
Stock mutual funds	Good way to get diversification; cheap way to have your funds managed.
Options	For suckers or professional investors. You are probably not the latter and hopefully not the former.
Commodity futures	For the gullible.
Stock-index futures	Have a role in sophisticated portfolio hedging strategies, which means they're not for you.
New issues	You don't pay commissions on new issues, which helps offset the loss most of them experience after you buy them.
Foreign stocks	There is always a bull market somewhere in the world. Difficult to evaluate, so use international mutual funds.
Precious metals	The only reason you should own a lot of gold is if you use it to fill teeth. Otherwise, no more than 5 to 10 percent of portfolio.
Collectibles	Nice to sit on, walk on, or look at. Don't expect to retire on the profits.
Interest-Earning Investments:	
Certificates of deposit	Generally lackluster returns after you finish giving Uncle Sam his piece of the interest. Chances are your local bank doesn't offer the best rates you can get, so shop around.

TYPE OF INVESTMENT	ASSESSMENT
Treasury securities	Yields fluctuate and usually become attractive once or twice per year. Safe, but how much safety do you need?
Mortgage-backed securities	Nice yields, but ever-present danger of getting back principal as interest rates drop.
Municipal bonds	Compare muni returns against after-tax returns on taxable securities. You may well find munis to be preferable.
Corporate bonds	Okay if you can get a much better yield than Treasuries. Otherwise, they don't justify the risk.
Junk bonds	Reserved for people who like high income and deteriorating principal.
Foreign fixed-income investments	Emerging investment area that is highly specialized and usually subjects you to currency risk. Buy through mutual funds only.
Fixed-income mutual funds	Good way to let someone else worry about the direction of interest rates. Offers diversification and inexpensive management.
Savings accounts	Better than nothing, but not much better. Keep only emergency funds there.
U.S. savings bonds	Nice gift; better than they used to be.
Money market funds	A temporary parking place only, please, since you can't beat inflation by very much on an after-tax basis. Money market mutual funds almost always beat bank money market accounts hands down.

Real Estate Investments:

Income-producing real estate	The average person's best route to wealth, if you buy at the right price and can stomach being a landlord.
Undeveloped land	An expensive little lot is better than a lot of cheap lots. In other words, 50 square feet in Manhattan, New York, is a better

TYPE OF INVESTMENT

ASSESSMENT

investment than 50 square miles in Manhattan, Montana.

Limited partnerships

Probably a good investment—next century. In the meantime, perhaps one deal in a hundred is worthwhile.

Any "new" investment that comes along; like "Unbundled Stock Units"

Excellent money-making opportunity, *if* you happen to be selling them to an unsuspecting public.

INVESTMENT ACTION PLAN

Current Status		
Needs Action	Okay or Not Applicable	
☐	☐	1. Establish realistic investment objectives and review/revise them periodically.
☐	☐	2. Make sure your investment objectives and planning recognize the economic outlook for your profession.
☐	☐	3. Become familiar with the variety of commonly used investment securities, and assess how each might be used in your investment portfolio.
☐	☐	4. Take advantage of any expertise you may have through your job experience that you may be able to apply to your investing.
☐	☐	5. List below the three worst shortcomings that you have that hinder or have hindered your investment success. The purpose of writing these down is to impress upon you that they should not be repeated.

1. _____
2. _____
3. _____

5

Taking the Pulse of
Your Investments

―

Now that you've set your reasonable investment goals, and have a basic idea of the various kinds of investments and the issues involved in investing, you're ready to learn how to choose the best investments for you and how to evaluate and control your portfolio, no matter how small (or large) it might be.

FOUR STEPS TO INVESTMENT SUCCESS

Since investing effectively is so important to your ultimate financial well-being, you need to develop a plan that will help guide you, both in deciding upon the types of investments to make and in reviewing your investments periodically. "Periodically" doesn't mean every day; otherwise, you'll become so concerned, you'll be likely to make investment changes too frequently. Rather, if you establish some sensible criteria now, you will be able to invest wisely and well without spending an inordinate amount of time worrying about your investments. The four steps to investment success are:

STEP ONE:
Deciding how much of your portfolio should be invested in stock, interest-earning investments, and perhaps, real estate.

STEP TWO:

Once you have decided how much of your investments should be in a given investment category, you need to determine whether you should purchase the securities directly, by buying individual stock and interest-earning securities, or indirectly, via mutual funds and limited partnerships.

STEP THREE:

Next, you need to determine within each category what classifications of investments might be appropriate—for example, for indirectly owned stocks, whether you should invest in aggressive growth stock mutual funds and/or international mutual funds.

STEP FOUR:

Finally, you need to select, carefully, specific investments within each category.

As you review the investment process, I will periodically refer to the Investment Allocation diagram that follows. It serves as the basis for your own investment decision making.

FIGURE 3

Investment Allocation

Method of Ownership	Investment Category		
	Stock	Interest-Earning	Real Estate
Direct Ownership			
Indirect Ownership (Mutual Fund/ Partnership)			

If you aren't quite sure what kinds of investments fit in each of the above boxes, they are listed and described in the Investment Bill of Fare that appears in the previous chapter. The following example shows how an appropriate investment portfolio can be put together.

Example: Rhea Bilitate, a therapist, has managed to set aside $25,000 over the past few years, which is now sitting in a money market account. She has just read the above "Four Steps to Investment Success" and is ready to invest her money more sensibly.

Step One: She decides that, while she may want to invest in real estate some time in the future, she doesn't have enough money yet, and therefore she should restrict her investments to stocks and interest-earning securities. She decides that 60 percent of her $25,000 or $15,000, should be invested in stocks, and 40 percent, or $10,000, should be invested in interest-earning securities.

Step One: Deciding on Proportion to Be Invested in Each Category

Method of Ownership	Investment Category		
	Stock	Interest-Earning	Real Estate
Direct Ownership			
Indirect Ownership (Mutual Fund/ Partnership)	60% ($15,000)	40% ($10,000)	0%

Step Two: Because her portfolio isn't very large yet—although she fully expects it will be eventually—she plans to invest most of her money in mutual funds. Nevertheless, she wants to become familiar with direct investing as well, so as indicated below, she is going to invest $5,000 in stocks and $3,000 in directly owned interest-earning investments.

Step Two: Deciding How Much to Invest Directly and Indirectly

Method of Ownership	Investment Category	
	Stock	Interest-Earning
Direct Ownership	$5,000	$3,000
Indirect Ownership (Mutual Fund/ Partnership)	$10,000	$7,000
Grand total:	$15,000	$10,000

Step Three: Rhea next needs to decide on the kinds of securities she will purchase within each of the four categories. After some deliberation, she has decided upon the investments that are indicated below.

Step Three: Deciding on Appropriate Kinds of Investments

Method of Ownership	Investment Category	
	Stock	Interest-Earning
Direct Ownership	High-quality growth stock $2,500 Blue chip stock 2,500 Total $5,000	Certificate of deposit $3,000 Total $3,000
Indirect Ownership (Mutual Fund/ Partnership)	Maximum capital-gains fund $3,000 Growth and income fund 5,000 International stock fund 2,000 Total $10,000	Government securities fund $4,000 Corporate bond fund 3,000 Total $7,000
Grand total:	$15,000	$10,000

Step Four: Rhea now needs to select specific investments for each of the categories that she has decided to invest in. We will leave that up to her, although she, as well as you, might benefit from the suggestions that follow.

The "four steps to investment success" are described below in more detail.

STEP ONE:

All too often, investors tend to invest in extremes. Even though you may think you have a well-balanced and well-diversified portfolio, you may be overlooking some kinds of investments that will help you achieve investment success. Therefore, before you do anything, you need to figure out how much of your total available investments (both now and in the future) should be invested in each of the three major investment categories (as described in Chapter 4): stocks, interest-earning investments, and real estate. Some people may not be interested in real estate, in which case the allocation is between stocks and interest-earning investments.

TIPS

■ The following guidelines will be helpful in determining the best way to allocate, or reallocate, your investments.

■ Younger and middle-aged people should weight their investments in favor of stocks, and if they are so inclined, real estate because these investments have the best chance of beating inflation and producing good long-term returns. However, some of the portfolio should probably remain conservatively invested. A typical investment allocation for younger people is 40 percent stock, 30 percent interest-earning investments, and 30 percent real estate (excluding the family home). Most people prefer not to invest in real estate. They might choose an allocation of 60 percent stock and 40 percent interest-earning investments or 50–50, which is perfectly okay and a lot easier to remember. Numerous studies of long-term stock and bond performance have indicated that a general portfolio mix of 50 to 60 percent stock and 40 to 50 percent interest-earning investments will provide very good long-term returns without taking too much risk.

■ Preretirees who are within about ten years of retirement should begin a gradual shift so that they increase the proportion of their money invested in more conservative securities. This tactic lessens the effects of being caught in a stock market downturn or real estate slump. Younger people have a longer "investment horizon" and can therefore weather the effects of a bear market better. If you, like most people, will need the portfolio to help meet living expenses, an appropriate pre-retirement investment mix might consist of 40 percent stocks and 60 percent interest-earning investments, or if you have real estate investments, 30 percent stock, 20 percent real estate, and 50 percent interest-earning investments.

■ Similarly, if you are retired, the amount of risk you can afford in your portfolio depends upon the extent to which you will have to rely on the funds to meet living expenses. Many retirees, of course, prefer investments that yield current income—either interest-earning securities or dividend-paying stocks. Since you also need capital appreciation to fund a (hopefully) long retirement, you should not abandon stocks entirely. Many retired medical professionals find that for the first time in their lives they have sufficient time to devote to stock market investing, and many do quite well at it.

Many medical professionals expect the future growth rate of their income to slow if not decline. Faced with this specter, some feel the need to increase the risk in their investments in the hope of obtaining a superior return. This is usually foolhardy. If you expect a slowing or a reversal in the growth rate of your income, you should factor that into your savings and investments projections and adjust your plans reasonably and accordingly. Adding risk to the portfolio to try to make up for the lower income is not an appropriate course of action.

■ Consider real estate on its economic merits, not its tax merits. For many people, real estate should be a component of a well-balanced portfolio, because its long term performance has been exceptional.

STEP TWO:

The second step involves deciding upon how much you want to have invested in directly owned securities like stocks and CDs and how much in indirectly owned securities like mutual funds. Most investors with small portfolios are best served by indirect investments, which provide diversification and professional management. As a general rule, the larger the portfolio, the larger the proportion that can be invested in directly owned stocks, bonds, and real estate.

TIPS

■ Direct investments have certain advantages and disadvantages. One of the major advantages is that you have control over the timing of capital gain recognition for tax purposes. In other words, as long as you hold on to a stock, interest-earning security, or real estate investment, you pay no taxes on its appreciation in value. Also, buying interest-earning investments and holding on to them until they mature avoids "interest-rate risk," which is the decline in the value of a bond if interest rates rise. Disadvantages of direct investments include the time and expense necessary to manage them effectively, particularly real estate. Also, there is usually less diversification in a portfolio of directly owned securities.

Medical professionals often accumulate portfolios of sufficient size that they can take advantage of certain investment strategies that are unavailable to people of lesser means. Some of these strategies, however, are too risky or too esoteric to be of use to any but a few investors. Other strategies, however, are worthwhile and should be considered in your investment planning. For example, you can write "covered-call stock options" to add additional income to an otherwise inactive stock portfolio. Covered-call writing entails selling stock options on stocks you already own, which if done regularly and monitored closely can add a 5 to 10 percent return on your stock investments, with little risk. Another strategy that may be of use involves donating low-cost basis shares to a charitable trust, as described in Chapter 8, in exchange for a lifetime income.

■ Indirect investments, consisting of mutual funds, and in the case of real estate, limited partnerships, have certain advantages and disadvantages as well. Advantages include greater diversification, professional management, and generally lower transaction costs. Disadvantages include the inability to control the timing of capital-gains tax realization, and with respect to bond mutual funds, exposure to possible interest-rate risk. In spite of the disadvantages, mutual funds belong in every portfolio. In fact, funds play a significant role in the investment strategies of professional investors with very large portfolios.

STEP THREE:

The third step in the investment allocation process breaks down the general categories of investment even further into specific industry, market, or fund categories. For example, if you feel that directly owned interest-earning investments belong in your portfolio, you have many to choose from, including munici-

---

The Greater Drool Theory

Stories of double-digit returns cause people to drool with envy. They in turn invest, causing the price of the security to rise, thereby increasing the level of drool of those people who haven't yet invested. At the peak, people are drooling so much that they slip (on their sputum), as does the price of the stock.

pal bonds, long-term CDs, Treasury securities, GNMA ("Ginnie Mae") certificates, and corporate bonds. Assuming, as is invariably the case, that you should also invest indirectly, via interest-earning mutual funds, you might consider, for example, municipal bond funds, corporate bond funds, and government securities funds.

TIP

Diversification is crucial. One of the most common mistakes that doctors and dentists make is putting too many eggs into one basket. It doesn't matter if it's a risky basket or a riskless basket. For example, some people are perfectly content putting all of their money in CDs. Over the long run they will suffer without diversification.

STEP FOUR:

The final step consists of selecting specific investments within each of the industry or fund categories—a particular bond or stock or mutual fund, for example. The following rules of thumb will help you select the right investments.

RULES OF THUMB FOR SELECTING INVESTMENTS

You will often be confronted with the pleasure and the dilemma of making investment decisions, including investing any dividend and interest income that is not automatically reinvested, your regular savings, and, perhaps, periodic windfalls, like an inheritance. By developing some informal guidelines you can simplify the process of investing—and of monitoring your investments.

STOCK INVESTMENTS are best made when stock prices in general are depressed. In other words: *buy low.* A readily available measure of relative stock prices is the price-earnings (P/E) ratio of a major market index, such as the Dow Jones Industrial Average. The P/E ratio is computed by dividing the market price of the

---

Buy stocks when no one else wants them; sell stocks when everyone else wants them.

stock by its earnings per share. A price-earnings ratio well above the historical average may indicate that the stock market is overpriced. For example, the Dow Jones Industrial P/E ratio reached twenty shortly before the October 1987 stock market crash. By way of comparison, the average Dow Jones Industrial P/E ratio over the past several years has been about fourteen. Investors may want to consider the current price-earnings ratios of the Dow Jones Industrial Average or Standard & Poor's 500 Stock Average in deciding whether or not to invest in stocks. If it is well above the historical average, avoid stocks. If below, consider stocks. The Dow Jones P/E ratio is available in *The Wall Street Journal* and *Barron's*.

TIP

Avoid following the crowd. Buy stocks of good companies that are currently out-of-favor on Wall Street. Also, participate in their dividend reinvestment programs, which not only automatically reinvest your dividends in more shares but also allow you to buy more shares of the company stock with no commission.

With respect to *interest-earning investments*, you may want to consider the bellwether yield on long-term Treasury bonds to judge how high or low interest rates are. Most interest rates move in tandem with the yield on long-term Treasury securities. In recent years, long-term Treasury yields around 9 percent have signaled attractive returns from interest-earning investments (particularly in tax-deferred retirement-oriented accounts). When the long-term Treasury yield exceeds 9 percent—as it has from time to time—you may wish to buy longer-term debt obligations or longer-term bond funds to lock in the high interest rates. If interest rates are low, you should buy shorter maturity interest-earning investments, such as money market funds or short-term CDs. Yields on interest-earning investments, including Treasury securities, are commonly available in the financial press.

TIP

When Treasury yields are high, pay particular attention to municipal bonds. Over the past several years, tax-exempt munis have been offering returns that are especially attractive when compared with the after-tax returns of their taxable brethren, such as corporate bonds, government-backed securities, and long-term CDs.

REAL ESTATE INVESTMENTS are especially difficult to evaluate, and doctors and dentists have earned a reputation, whether deserved or not, of selecting them particularly poorly. If, for example, you happened to purchase a pre-tax-reform real estate limited partnership solely for its tax advantages, and you are still stuck with it, you're probably not terribly pleased. Be patient. You can save those passive losses, and deduct them from passive income at any time in the future. Evaluate a prospective real estate investment as you would any other investment. Weigh its tax ramifications, but remember that they are only one aspect of its overall financial viability, and a minor one at that.

Medical professionals are favorite targets of real estate limited partnership salespeople. The vast majority of these deals are mediocre at best. Avoid making real estate limited partnership investments unless you are thoroughly familiar with and trust the people who are selling the investment, and unless you are willing to thoroughly evaluate (or have a knowledgeable person such as your accountant or lawyer evaluate) the offering memorandum.

Even many experienced investors feel intimidated by real estate investments. Luckily, there are a couple of rules of thumb that can help you assess the financial viability of an investment in income-producing real estate, whether you are buying the property yourself or investing in a limited partnership. The simpler rule involves comparing the total selling price with the current gross annual rental. A property that is selling for much more than seven times gross annual rental is likely to yield a negative cash flow. For example, if a duplex selling for $180,000 generates $15,000 in annual rent, it is selling at twelve times annual rental. The rent probably won't cover the mortgage, property taxes, insurance, and all the other costs of being a landlord, so you'll probably have to pour more cash into the investment. If you put a sizable cash down payment into the property to assure a positive cash flow, you're only fooling yourself, because there's an opportunity cost associated with tying up a lot of cash in real estate that could otherwise be earning interest.

Similarly, if you're considering a real estate limited partnership investment where the general partner pays more than

---

The key to saving the money necessary to build up your investments: Spend the same amount of money during the three days *after* payday as you do during the three days *before* payday.

Typical Doctor/Dentist's $500,000 Investment Portfolio:

	Annual Rate of Return	
	Expected	*Actual*
$200,000 in dry oil well limited partnerships	35%	unknown
$100,000 in Texas and Florida real estate limited partnerships with single-digit occupancy rates	35%	unknown
$100,000 in a recently delisted stock of a company that owns a chain of video-game arcades	35%	unknown
$100,000 in checking account	0%	0%

seven times gross annual rental to buy a property, the partnership is paying too much, unless it can reasonably expect a dramatic increase in the value of the property—if the partnership is planning an immediate condo conversion, for example. Of course, the general partner, and more particularly, the salespeople, always expect great things out of the deal although, alas, a less optimistic prognosis would often be more accurate.

The second real estate rule of thumb is to calculate the capitalization rate, usually referred to as the "cap rate." The formula is simple:

$$\text{Capitalization rate} = \frac{\text{Net operating income}}{\text{Total amount invested}}$$

"Total amount invested" includes both the down payment and borrowed money necessary to buy the property. "Net operating income" is total rental income—allowing for vacancies—less all expenses except debt service. For example, a limited partnership in an apartment building requiring a total investment of $3,500,000 has an estimated net operating income of $300,000.

The cap rate is $300,000 divided by $3,500,000, or 8.6 percent. A cap rate of eight or greater is considered desirable. Whether you are investing in real estate yourself or through a limited partnership, make sure the numbers are realistic. A favorite trick of real estate agents and general partners is known as "bumping to market"—raising rent projections from what they currently are to a supposed market level in order to make the deal look more attractive. If you've ever looked for rental property as an investment, you've probably heard the real estate agent say, "the rents are this low only because the tenants have been in there so long. All you have to do is evict these old folks and rent the apartments to yuppies." Unless you take great pleasure in evicting elderly people, you should respond: "Tell the current owner to kick them out. When the building is full of tenants paying reasonable rents, I'll be ready to negotiate."

Undeveloped land is particularly difficult to evaluate. Generally, land with significant appreciation potential is well situated and, therefore, very expensive. Cheap land usually remains cheap. Don't think you've spotted something that everybody else, including all the experts, has overlooked. Real estate investing continues to be an excellent way to create wealth, but those who are successful at it share one characteristic—patience. When, based on the above parameters, they find that real estate is overpriced, they are happy to wait until market conditions make a purchase feasible.

Medical professionals usually lack the time—and many lack the managerial skills—necessary to purchase, maintain, and manage income-producing real estate investments effectively. Avoid making major commitments to income-producing real estate until you gain experience (or your spouse gains experience) in handling smaller properties. Real estate investing provides marvelous wealth creation possibilities, but on the other hand, it can result in mental and fiscal duress.

CASH EQUIVALENT INVESTMENTS

You may be wondering what you should do with your money if:

1. You think stock prices are too high, and
2. You think interest rates are too low, and

The eventual performance of an investment is inversely related to the enthusiasm exuded by the individual who wants to sell it to you.

---

3. You are either uninterested in real estate or can't find any attractively priced real estate.

You don't have to put the cash in your mattress. Instead, you can park your money in what are known as "cash equivalent" investments, which are really just very short-term interest-earning investments. Cash equivalents should generally be viewed as a temporary place to invest your money when market conditions, as *you* define them, aren't favorable. Cash equivalents include money market funds, Treasury bills, and short-term CDs. Cash-equivalent investments should be viewed only as temporary, because they do not offer any hope of beating inflation by very much after you finish paying taxes on the interest. Nevertheless, there are times when cash equivalents are certainly a preferable investment until stock market, interest rate, or real estate conditions become more favorable.

DECIDING WHEN TO SELL

While cash-equivalent investments should be sold when you can find a more attractive investment opportunity, deciding when to sell your other investments is a more difficult problem. First of all, you shouldn't make any investment with the intention of selling it within the next few years. One of the reasons you buy high quality stocks, interest-earning investments, and mutual funds is to avoid having to worry all the time about whether or not you should sell them. Nevertheless, you will probably end up investing in some dogs along the way. I use the following rule: If I am disappointed in the performance of the investment over two consecutive years, I'll usually sell it. I define "disappointing" as a stock that does not keep up with the Standard & Poor's 500 Stock Average over two consecutive years, and a mutual fund that lags the annual average performance of its category for two consecutive years. In other words, if I own a growth and income mutual fund that underperforms the annual average performance for all growth and income mutual funds for two consecutive years, it's history. Perhaps this rule of thumb means that I will hold on to a lousy investment longer than I should, but I'd rather make that mistake than make the mistake of selling too often. I *know* that selling too often will not work.

PORTFOLIO REDEPLOYMENT

If you follow my suggestion and maintain a relatively fixed proportion of investment in stocks, interest-earning securities, and perhaps, real estate, you may have to redeploy some of these investments periodically in order to maintain this proportion.

Example: Dr. Bruno Brace, an orthodontist, has $40,000 in investments. He invested the money a year ago by placing $20,000 in stock mutual funds and the other $20,000 in a Treasury bill and a couple of bond funds. Over the past year, the stock market has increased rather markedly while the bond market has been so-so. He just summarized his portfolio and found that the stock side had increased to $25,000 in the past year while the bond side is now worth $21,000. So, Dr. Brace's total portfolio is now $46,000. He should maintain a fifty–fifty split between stocks and interest-earning securities, so he should sell $2,000 of his stock mutual funds and purchase $2,000 of interest-earning securities to bring him back to an even allocation ($23,000 in stocks and $23,000 in interest-earning investments). Note that by periodically summarizing, and if necessary, redeploying his investments, Dr. Brace is forced to "do the right thing." In other words, he sells some of his stock portfolio after it has increased in value (this is "selling high") and buys interest-earning securities after they have experienced a lackluster year ("buying low"). Had stocks declined in value, Dr. Brace would have been buying stocks to bring the stock side back up to his desired allocation percentage. Most investors do the opposite—they buy stocks when they are high and sell them when they are low.

AVOIDING INVESTMENT OVERLOAD

While you should always keep in mind the need to maintain an appropriately balanced portfolio—one that is allocated in accordance with your wishes, you don't want to go overboard just because you find market conditions to be irresistible. For example, even if stocks appear cheap, you may be ill-advised to invest additional money in stocks if you already have a high percentage of your total portfolio in stocks.

SELECTING AND MANAGING YOUR INVESTMENT ADVISERS

Some physicians and dentists are perfectly content to make their own investment decisions, and can manage very well by using discount brokers and/or no-load mutual funds. The majority, however, are counseled by one or more investment advisers. Investment advisers range from commission-based stockbrokers and insurance agents to fee-based investment advisers and managers. I have intentionally omitted another commonly utilized class of investment adviser, usually referred to as the "hot tipster" and normally assuming the role of golf or bridge partner.

Most medical professionals are advised by stockbrokers. Unfortunately, too few of them take the time to carefully choose their broker(s). That's why you receive so many cold calls from brokers. Sadly, this is a frequent method of selecting a broker. Taking the time to research a brokerage firm and broker will pay off in the long run. Select a firm and broker that are experienced in the type of investments that interest you. I have worked very well with brokers who are specialized in certain areas—stocks, Treasury securities, municipal bonds, or covered option writing. I prefer brokers who have been in the business for many years. Since they have survived all kinds of market adversity, they are probably good at what they do. They also probably have numerous accounts and therefore don't have to extract big commissions off my hide to keep food on their tables. Once you sign up a broker, recognize that good advice doesn't always make money, and when it does make money, it may not make a lot. The single most important thing for you to do is to *manage* the relationship. I saw the account a few years ago of a dentist who had given his broker carte blanche trading authorization on a $150,000 account. The result for the dentist: an 80 percent diminution in value in one year when the market overall was up! The result for the broker: over $20,000 in commissions. No matter how busy you are, you must participate in each investment decision. If you are too busy to do so, you need an experienced investment adviser or manager who will take over the chore of managing your money on a day-to-day basis.

Investment advisers and managers may—but not always—alleviate the conflict of interest that is inherent in broker-client relationships because they are paid either on a fee-for-service basis or as a percentage of assets under management. Unfortunately, you have to have several hundred thousand dollars of investable funds to receive the quality of counsel you deserve. In addition, selection of an investment adviser or manager is no easy task. The first requirement is that the firm be able to accommodate your specific investment objectives. Be sure to check individual performance records through both bull and bear markets. Compare fees, services, size, and investment philosophies of several different companies. Interview the managers. Like any

---

Pond's Law of Investment Return Proportionality:

The rate of return that someone boasts about on a recent investment is equal to the number of losing investments that preceded this "fantastic" investment. For example, if your crony boasts that he just got a 51 percent return on a hot stock, his previous 51 investments ended up losing money.

investment decision, it is better to spread your money among two or more investment advisers, but this requires that you have a lot of money in your till. Just as with a broker, once you have made your decision, don't try to second-guess the manager. These relationships *must* be evaluated over a multiyear period. This doesn't mean that you don't need to pay attention to them now. Keep informed about your portfolio, and manage your investment manager. If you have specific orders for your investment manager, make them. I'm acquainted with a surgeon who is extremely knowledgeable about developments in his field that emanate from young, publicly traded medical instrument companies. His retirement fund investment managers do not hesitate to follow his instructions to add or delete these stocks from his portfolio.

If, on the other hand, you want to manage your own investments, there is an abundance of good information that can help you be an effective long-term investor. Most libraries have the *Value Line Investment Survey,* the bible for stock investors, and the *Wiesenberger Investment Companies Service,* the bible for mutual fund investors. *Barron's,* the weekly newspaper for investors, also contains a wealth of timely information. Finally, just reading the business and personal finance section of your local newspaper will help you learn more about investing, and current market conditions. Whether you do it yourself, rely on stockbrokers, or do a little of both, take some time to learn more about investing. You will be well rewarded for the effort.

Medical professionals often fail to take advantage of their professional expertise in their investment decisions. Do not hesitate to make investments in areas where you have an advantage by virtue of your professional expertise. Often, this may involve emerging companies in the medical or drug business. Of course, any such investments, particularly in newer companies or nascent technologies, should be limited in relation to your total investment portfolio.

Averaging down to the poorhouse: If your broker urges you to buy more shares of a stock that has lost value in order to "average down," tell him to let you know when the price of the stock reaches zero so that you can buy the whole company for nothing.

Remember, nothing in financial planning should be viewed as an "either/or" decision. Even if the bulk of your portfolio is or will be professionally managed, you will probably have at least some money in a brokerage account and some money that you manage yourself. This is fine, but don't needlessly complicate your life (not to mention your tax preparer's life) by having numerous accounts. Speaking of tax preparers, always bear in mind that your investments are likely to affect other areas of financial planning, such as income taxes, estate planning, and retirement planning. It is crucial that you review your portfolio periodically with your other advisers.

The next section will illustrate how you can put together a good long-term investment portfolio that will help you achieve financial security.

PUTTING TOGETHER AN ALL-WEATHER INVESTMENT PORTFOLIO

We've said a lot about structuring an investment portfolio and selecting appropriate investments. Now we can look at how this might be done in real life. Incidentally, the same principles apply to both small and large portfolios, so the following illustrations will take you from a $1,000 portfolio to a $500,000 portfolio. All of the illustrations, except for the $500,000 portfolio, assume that the investor wants to maintain an allocation of 50 percent stock investments and 50 percent interest-earning investments, which, by the way, isn't a bad split for most of us.

THE $1,000 PORTFOLIO—JUST THE BEGINNING

What, a $1,000 investment portfolio? Why not? Unless you're some kind of heir, everyone starts at the bottom. There's no reason why you shouldn't begin to develop good habits by investing your $1,000 much like a pension manager handles a multimillion-dollar portfolio. The rules are the same.

You can start out by putting $500 into a growth and income stock mutual fund and $500 into a government securities fund. Incidentally, there are many good mutual funds that have investment minimums of $500 or less. Alternatively, you could invest the $1,000 in a "balanced" mutual fund, which consists of both stock and interest-earning securities. The $1,000 portfolio is presented below.

SAMPLE $1,000 Portfolio

Method of Ownership	Investment Category	
	Stock	Interest-Earning
Direct Ownership		
Indirect Ownership (Mutual Fund/ Partnership)	Growth and income fund $500	Government securities fund $500

THE $10,000 PORTFOLIO—PASSING THROUGH

When you have $10,000 to invest, you can begin to expand your horizons somewhat, although you will still probably want to restrict your holdings to mutual funds, and perhaps a CD. You aren't quite at a level where you can start to make direct investments. But don't fret, because there are a lot of good mutual funds that will help you meet your investment objectives.

SAMPLE $10,000 Portfolio

Method of Ownership	Investment Category	
	Stock	Interest-Earning
Direct Ownership		
Indirect Ownership (Mutual Fund/ Partnership)	Aggressive growth fund $2,000	Government securities fund $3,000
	Growth and income fund 3,000	Corporate bond fund 2,000
	Total $5,000	Total $5,000

As the following table shows, you can divide your portfolio among several mutual funds, and the funds will provide diversification as well as professional management of your hard-earned savings.

THE $100,000 PORTFOLIO—GETTING THERE

Once your portfolio exceeds $20,000 or so, you can begin to make directly owned investments in stock and interest-earning securities. The following table shows how a $100,000 portfolio might be structured so that $25,000 is invested in each of the four categories, thereby maintaining a fifty–fifty split between total stock investments and total interest-earning investments. The directly owned stocks box includes $5,000 in each of five high-quality stocks. Most of the dividend-paying companies that you would want to invest in have dividend reinvestment programs. Be sure to participate in them so that your dividend checks can be used to purchase more stocks.

SAMPLE $100,000 Portfolio

Method of Ownership	Investment Category	
	Stock	Interest-Earning
Direct Ownership	$5,000 in each of five high quality blue chip stocks and growth stocks Total $25,000	CD $5,000 Municipal bonds 10,000 Corporate bonds 10,000 Total $25,000

Indirect Ownership (Mutual Fund/ Partnership)	Aggressive
	  growth fund $5,000
	Growth and
	  income fund 10,000
	International
	  fund 5,000
	Gold fund 5,000
	  Total $25,000
		Government
		  securities
		  fund $10,000
		Municipal
		  bond fund 10,000
		Corporate
		  bond fund 5,000
		  Total $25,000

The larger portfolio allows you to invest in a wider range of securities. Note that the stock mutual funds component now includes investments in an international fund and a gold fund.

THE $500,000 PORTFOLIO—JUST WHAT THE DOCTOR ORDERED

In addition to making more of the same investments you made for your first $100,000, when your portfolio exceeds $100,000, you can begin to consider a number of additional

SAMPLE $500,000 Portfolio

Method of Ownership	Investment Category		
	Stock	Interest-Earning	Real Estate
Direct Ownership	$10,000 in each of ten common stock investments Total $100,000	CDs $25,000 Municipal bonds 25,000 Treasury notes 25,000 Corporate bonds 25,000 Total $100,000	
Indirect Ownership (Mutual Fund/ Partnership)	Aggressive growth funds $20,000 Growth and income funds 30,000 International funds 25,000 Gold fund 25,000 Total $100,000	Government securities funds $25,000 Municipal bond funds 25,000 Corporate bond funds 25,000 Deferred annuity 25,000 Total $100,000	Two to four real estate limited partnerships* Total $100,000

*Alternatively, investment in directly owned real estate could be made.

investments, including more speculative stocks and stock mutual funds, individual purchases of government securities and mortgage-backed securities, income-producing real estate, undeveloped land, and real estate limited partnerships. Tax-deferred annuities, which are discussed in Chapter 7, may also play a role in a larger portfolio. The diagram illustrates a well-balanced $500,000 portfolio, which includes some real estate investments.

ON THE ROAD TO INVESTMENT RECOVERY

At this stage, you're probably ready to take some steps to evaluate your investments, and if necessary, prescribe some preventive medicine and some corrective surgery.

First, find out where you stand. Summarize all your investments. Your most important investment, your home, if you own one, doesn't count for purposes of this analysis. Be sure to include all funds invested in any retirement plans that require you to control where the funds are invested, such as IRAs and 401(k) plans. An Investment Summary work sheet is provided to help you take inventory.

Second, decide what changes, if any, need to be made to your current investments. Are they concentrated too much in a single investment category? If so, you should plan to redeploy the investments to achieve a better diversified portfolio. Redeployment doesn't need to happen overnight, but start to think about a timetable. An Investment Allocation Analysis is provided to help you plan your redeployment.

Third, begin to invest more money, according to your overall plan and according to those rules of thumb that will help you achieve your investment objectives. *If you haven't been saving enough, start doing so immediately.*

Finally, review your investments periodically, but not too often. If you make the right investments initially, there is no need to monitor their performance constantly. Most successful individual investors review their investments only once every few months at most.

If you follow these guidelines, you will probably end up with a duller portfolio. You won't have much to brag about. Your cronies will probably make you feel inferior because they will go on making sexy investments that, once in a while, produce a

Investment Summary Work Sheet

This work sheet can be used to facilitate the often laborious process of summarizing your investment portfolio. Date at which market values are indicated: _____

Description	Number of Shares or Face Value	Date Acquired	Original Cost	Current Market Value	Estimated Annual Interest or Dividend
1. Cash equivalent investments:					
Money market funds and accounts					
_____	_____	_____	$_____	$_____	$_____
_____	_____	_____	_____	_____	_____
_____	_____	_____	_____	_____	_____
Savings Accounts					
_____	_____	_____	_____	_____	_____
_____	_____	_____	_____	_____	_____
_____	_____	_____	_____	_____	_____
CDs					
_____	_____	_____	_____	_____	_____
_____	_____	_____	_____	_____	_____
_____	_____	_____	_____	_____	_____
Other cash equivalent investments					
_____	_____	_____	_____	_____	_____
Total cash equivalent investments			$_____	$_____	$_____
2. Fixed-income investments:					
U.S. government securities					
_____	_____	_____	$_____	$_____	$_____
_____	_____	_____	_____	_____	_____
U.S. government securities funds					
_____	_____	_____	_____	_____	_____
_____	_____	_____	_____	_____	_____
Mortgage-backed securities					
_____	_____	_____	_____	_____	_____
_____	_____	_____	_____	_____	_____

Description	Number of Shares or Face Value	Date Acquired	Original Cost	Current Market Value	Estimated Annual Interest or Dividend
Mortgage-backed securities funds					
Corporate bonds					
Corporate bond funds					
Municipal bonds					
Municipal bond funds					
Other fixed-income investments					
Total fixed-income investments			$	$	$

3. **Equity investments:**
Common stock in publicly traded companies

Description	Number of Shares or Face Value	Date Acquired	Original Cost	Current Market Value	Estimated Annual Interest or Dividend
			$	$	$
Stock mutual funds					
Precious metals and precious metal funds					
Other equity investments					
Total equity investments			$	$	$

Description	Number of Shares or Face Value	Date Acquired	Original Cost	Current Market Value	Estimated Annual Interest or Dividend
4. Real estate investments: Undeveloped land					
			$_____	$_____	$_____
Directly owned, income-producing real estate					
Real estate limited partnerships					
Total real estate investments			$_____	$_____	$_____
5. Interests in privately held businesses:			$_____	$_____	$_____
Total interests in privately held businesses			$_____	$_____	$_____
Grand total investments			$_____	$_____	$_____

boastworthy return. But the way to win in this business is to devise a reasonable investment program that meets your unique needs, and stick to it. When you're retired, do your cronies a favor and buy them dinner at a nice restaurant. *You'll* be able to afford it.

INVESTMENT ALLOCATION ANALYSIS

This work sheet allows you to view the percentage allocation of your total portfolio versus your desired or "target" allocation. Transfer the current market value totals for each investment category from the Investment Summary into the first two columns below. Then calculate the percent of your total investment portfolio in each category. Compare these percentages with your desired portfolio allocation, which can be entered in the right column. This analysis should be prepared at least annually.

Date at which market values are indicated: _____

Investment Category	Current Market Value			Percent of Portfolio	Target Percent of Portfolio
	Personal Investments	Retirement-Plan Investments*	Total		
Stock	$.....	$.....	$.....	.....%	.....%
Interest-earning investments	.....	.....	.....	......	.....
Real estate	.....	.....	.....	.....	.....
Grand total	.....	.....	.....	100%	100%

Comments: _____
_____
_____
_____
_____

*List all retirement-plan investments in which you control the investment allocations, including IRA and 401(k) plans.

INVESTMENT MANAGEMENT ACTION PLAN

Current Status		
Needs Action	Okay or Not Applicable	
☐	☐	1. Summarize all your investments, including any retirement-plan investments that you manage.
☐	☐	2. Determine how your investments are allocated, in total, among the three investment categories: stock, interest-earning, and real estate.
☐	☐	3. Plan how you are going to redeploy your investments to achieve a more appropriate allocation.
☐	☐	4. Begin, if you haven't already, to save at regular intervals in order to build up your investment portfolio.

Current Status		
Needs Action	Okay or Not Applicable	
☐	☐	5. If your income is likely to fluctuate, adjust your saving and investing to assure that sufficient resources to meet living expenses will be available.
☐	☐	6. Spend at least some time learning about investments and the current investment climate.
☐	☐	7. Review the status of your portfolio periodically.
☐	☐	8. Coordinate your investing with other areas of financial planning, particularly taxes and estate planning, but don't let the desire to save taxes dominate your investing.
☐	☐	9. Recognize that a buy-and-hold strategy is almost always the most beneficial way to manage a personal portfolio.
☐	☐	10. Mutual funds should play a role in every portfolio, preferably no-load funds.
☐	☐	11. While real estate is often a sound long-term investment, never invest in a property that violates general guidelines outlined in the chapter.
☐	☐	12. Select and control your investment advisers carefully.
☐	☐	13. Above all, be consistent in carrying out your investment objectives.

INVESTMENT ALLOCATION PLANNER

It's now time for you to plan how you should allocate your investments, just as it's been done in the chapter. If you don't yet have any investments, you can still plan for the day when you will, because that day (hopefully) won't be far off.

Investment Category

Method of Ownership	Stock	Interest-Earning	Real Estate
Direct Ownership			
Indirect Ownership (Mutual Fund/ Partnership)			

Comments:_____
_____
_____
_____

Investment "To Do" List:_____
_____
_____
_____

6 | Minimizing Your Income-Tax Extractions

Figuring out ways to save on taxes is as American as apple pie and baseball. I never cease to be amazed by how obsessed people are with dreaming up elaborate schemes to avoid paying taxes. The law has consistently upheld this American right. In the words of Judge Learned Hand: "Over and over again, courts have said that there is nothing sinister in so arranging one's affairs as to keep taxes as low as possible. Everybody does so, rich or poor; and all do right, for nobody owes any public duty to pay more tax than the law demands; taxes are enforced exactions, not voluntary contributions."

But just because there are legal ways to pay Uncle Sam less, that does not mean those options are always preferable. How many billions of dollars have been invested over the past decade in tax-sheltered limited partnerships that have proven worthless? Tax planning is an important part of personal financial planning, but *it is just one part.* Any investment or financial decision should include an evaluation of its tax ramifications, but none should be regarded solely or even primarily on that basis. There are many cases in which the option that results in a lower cut for Uncle Sam also results in a lower cut for you! Other tax-saving strategies simply aren't worth the effort, or may end up backfiring.

Example: Dr. Bogart, a city health officer, never even knew he had a great-aunt Mae until her estate administrators wrote to inform him that she had left him $20,000. The Bogarts were beginning to become concerned about how they would pay for their children's education, so they figured this money could be used for those costs. "I'm not going to let taxes eat up my kids' college tuition," said Dr. Bogart, so he decided to do as several of his colleagues had done and gift the money to his oldest child, who had just turned fourteen. He knew that by so doing he would not be subject to the "kiddie tax" on this money and the income, therefore, would be taxed at the son's low rate. "At last," the Bogarts thought, "we're able to shelter some of the income from taxes."

But how much do they save? In fact, they'll be lucky to save $300 per year in taxes, and this strategy could end up backfiring. By transferring the money to the child, the Bogarts could end up qualifying for less financial aid than they would have had the money been retained in the parents' names, because financial-aid authorities expect the child's resources to be exhausted to pay for college costs, but not the parents'. Another potential pitfall is what happens if the child decides to eschew or postpone college? They can't get their money back. This may be a particular risk in the Bogarts' case because their son, Humphrey, is obsessed with the movie business and keeps threatening to run away to Hollywood.

Surprising as it may seem, many doctors behave like Dr. Bogart. Doctors, maybe because of their high incomes, are traditionally too preoccupied with minimizing their tax burden. Tax shelters are not very useful in the current tax environment, since taxes aren't taking the huge bite they did formerly. But taxes still manage to nibble up enough income to be a nuisance. Good tax planning takes a lot of the sting out of the bite. However, good tax planning cannot be accomplished between Thanksgiving and Christmas each year.

The purpose of this chapter is to help you identify certain strategies and rules that benefit medical professionals. Doctors, dentists, and other health-care employees tend to be guided by grandiose tax-saving schemes, which often lack economic substance—in spite of what the colorful brochures tell you. Many busy and affluent health-care professionals also rely too heavily

---

If you're so mad about paying so much in income taxes, quit working. Your tax bill will plummet.

on their tax preparers, who, while they may provide you with sound advice, are obviously not as familiar with your own needs as you are, particularly over the long term. In fact, effective tax planning often takes years to accomplish. One final note: The Tax "Complification" Act of 1986 reduced the marginal tax rates so significantly that tax shelters are no longer a significant issue. Things were a lot different when you were taxed at 40 or 50 cents on the dollar, but many medical professionals still haven't realized the changes in thinking that are required for the current income-tax-rate environment. The more you ask, "What is the income-tax impact of this transaction?" the more likely you are to become so tax-driven that you literally sacrifice income.

TAX ISSUES PERTAINING TO HEALTH-CARE PROFESSIONALS

TAX DEFERRAL

Tax deferral, most often in the form of retirement-oriented accounts, is an important tax-advantaged investment alternative for health-care professionals—even those who work for organizations that already have pension plans. Many of them are designed to force you to save, or at least strongly discourage you from spending, because if you contribute money to them, it accumulates with no tax liability until it is withdrawn; whereas if you withdraw it prematurely, it incurs stiff penalties. In addition, when you contribute to some of these plans, you can deduct the amount you contribute from your current earnings. Chapter 7, which deals with retirement planning, contains explanations of tax-deferred retirement plans and investments. If it's hard to choose between them, don't worry. You can set up as many as you can afford. The one thing you do sacrifice is liquidity, so you really shouldn't put any funds in these accounts that you might need before retirement. To sum up my feelings on tax-deferred investing, anyone with earned income should establish an individual retirement account (IRA), anyone with any income from self-employment should contribute to a self-employed retirement account such as a Keogh or simplified employee pension (SEP) plan, and anyone whose employer offers a pension plan should be sure to participate to the maximum.

With all of the confusion generated by the tax reform of the 1980s (there were seven major pieces of tax legislation enacted during the decade), we often tend to lose sight of the fact that Congress retained intact the one tax shelter that, in my experience, has been responsible for the vast majority of family wealth accumulation in this country. We can still buy and hold capital assets free of taxation on the unrealized accretion in value. In English, this means you can buy stock and real estate, and so long as you hold on to it, you will not pay any capital gains taxes on the increase in its value. Time and time again, as I have reviewed the portfolios of some very wealthy families, I find the same pattern. They either bought a lot of real estate and have held on, to it for many, many years, or they bought a lot of common stock and have held on to it for many, many years. The annual returns they have enjoyed on these long-held investments are often 20 percent, 30 percent, or more of their original cost basis. Why? Because, in the instance of real estate, they have been able to increase rents and, over time, have reduced operating expenses and reduced, if not eliminated, mortgage payments. In the instance of stocks, these families have invested in blue chip stocks of good companies with strong dividend-paying records (I refer to them as "the Generals," like Electric and Motors), and these companies increase their dividend rates over the years. Mind you, all of this has been enjoyed without any payment of capital gains tax. This is wealth creation at its best, and there is no reason why you can't do the same thing. As the saying goes, "One way to get rich is to look at what rich people do, and do the same thing." While I don't want you to spend like rich people, we will both be delighted if you invest like rich people.

Remember Judge Learned Hand's comment on choosing the method of completing a transaction that will result in the lowest tax burden? One of the easiest ways to do this is to decide when you want to pay certain tax-deductible bills and when you want to receive certain income, on the basis of how it will affect your tax liability. The transaction remains fundamentally the same—all you change is the timing, but timing can have a big effect on your tax bill. One commonly used technique to postpone the receipt of income is to defer billing for services performed in December until the very end of the month, so the payment is likely to be received in January. You have to be careful of the "constructive receipt" rule, however, which treats any amount that is subject to the taxpayer's unqualified demand as taxable income, whether or not it has actually been received in cash.

DEDUCTIONS

Income-tax deductions can reduce your immediate burden, but once again, don't get carried away, and don't let tax considerations cloud your better judgment. It's good to know what expenses are tax-deductible, and to what extent, so that you don't overlook anything in April, but it's usually not good to let deductibility determine how you spend.

You can probably get the most mileage out of business-expense deductions. Most health-care professionals incur numerous expenses that are considered deductible ordinary and necessary expenses incurred in the practice of a profession. Deductible expenses include the cost of supplies; expense of operating and maintaining an automobile used in making professional calls; dues paid to professional societies; rent paid for office rooms; cost of fuel, light, water, and telephone used in the office; the cost of hiring assistants; and the cost of books, instruments, and equipment when such items have a short useful life. The cost of items with a long useful life, like office furniture and equipment and medical books, cannot be deducted in the year purchased; instead, they are depreciated over several years. Expenses incurred in attending business conventions and the costs of subscriptions to professional journals or information services bought in connection with the performance of your professional duties are normally deductible as a business expense, and so are contributions to qualified pension plans. A member of the medical profession is allowed a deduction for business entertainment, as long as there is a direct relationship between the expense and the development or expansion of a medical practice. However, a doctor's staff privilege fee paid to a hospital is a nondeductible capital expenditure.

If you are considering establishing or buying a practice, discuss with a qualified accountant or lawyer how the form of the business will affect the deductibility of certain expenses. For example, if the business is incorporated, otherwise nondeductible personal expenditures, such as life insurance premiums, may be deductible as a corporate business expense for officer-shareholders. Other expenses are affected by the form of business as well. Medical malpractice insurance is a particularly interesting case. A self-employed doctor may deduct the premium costs of malpractice insurance, but a doctor who is employed by someone else (like a hospital) can only deduct the premiums as an itemized deduction. Whether malpractice premiums paid to a physician-owned insurance carrier are deductible depends on how the carrier is organized.

A doctor or dentist may depreciate part of the purchase price of a medical practice, if he or she can show buying a wasting asset, such as patients' records, the useful life and value of which can be estimated. Similarly, a doctor may be able to deduct payment for the right to practice in a hospital over his or her life expectancy.

Educational expenses may be deductible business expenses if certain conditions are met. The expenses are deductible if the education maintains or improves skills required in the professional's trade or business or meets the express requirements of the professional's employer. If the educational expenses meet these requirements, reimbursements by the employer to the employee do not need to be reported by the employee-professional and such reimbursements are not considered wages for purposes of Social Security taxes, unemployment taxes, or income-tax withholding. However, if the education being sought is a minimum educational requirement for qualification in a profession or part of a program of study that will lead to qualifying an individual for a new profession, trade, or business, expenditures are not deductible. Moreover, for the education to be considered as maintaining or improving professional skills, you must be engaged in the profession at the time you take the course; merely being a member in good standing is not enough. Only educational expenses incurred for a nonadvanced degree under a reimbursement or other expense allowance arrangement with the employer are fully deductible. If full reimbursement is not made, the unreimbursed portion of the educational expense is allowable only as a miscellaneous itemized deduction, subject to the 2 percent floor.

Sometimes it's hard to tell which courses improve skills in your medical field and which courses train you for a new trade. The IRS allows general practitioners to deduct the cost of short refresher courses, even when the courses relate to specialized fields. These courses maintain or improve skills and do not qualify the doctor for a new profession. A practicing psychiatrist

---

An impossible dream: Preparing a tax return without having a single argument with your spouse.

may deduct the cost of attending an accredited psychoanalytic institute to qualify to practice psychoanalysis. A social worker was allowed a deduction for the cost of psychoanalysis, and in one case, a psychiatrist was allowed to deduct the cost of personal therapy sessions conducted through telephone conversations and tape cassettes. The court decided the therapy improved his job skills by eliminating psychological blind spots that prevented him from understanding his patients' problems. A licensed practical nurse may not deduct the costs of a college program that qualifies him or her as a "physician's assistant," which is a new job. The two professions are subject to different registration and certification requirements under state law, and the physician's assistant may perform duties, such as physical examinations and minor surgery, that go beyond practical nursing duties.

INCOME OF INTERNS AND RESIDENTS

Payments received by interns and resident physicians are generally considered taxable compensation, even though training and experience are gained while working. In a few cases, however, residents' grants are treated as tax-free fellowships.

TAX-EXEMPT INVESTMENTS

Tax-exempt investments can still be a smart way to invest, but they are subject to the same principles by which you would evaluate any other investment. Over the past several years, the yield on many long-term tax-exempt bonds has not been much less than the yield offered by taxable long-term Treasury bonds. When you consider that you don't have to pay federal income tax on the interest, tax-exempt bonds begin to look like a pretty good addition to a diversified investment portfolio. For example, an investor in the 31 percent federal tax bracket would have to earn almost 12 percent on a taxable bond to match an 8 percent tax-exempt yield on an after-tax basis. Single-state municipals (or municipal obligations of Puerto Rico) can provide exemption from both federal and state income taxes. An alternative to buy-

---

Death is tough to postpone. Income taxes, however, can be postponed by filing an extension.

ing individual municipal issues is to invest in municipal bond mutual funds and unit investment trusts that offer tax-free compounding, diversification, and professional securities selection for a low price.

Tax-exempt bonds are one of the few alternatives left that protect current income from taxes and are still generally a good investment, but you must be careful to weigh your alternative minimum tax position before investing in them. The interest on some municipal bond issues that are used to finance activities that are not related to the issuing government are subject to the AMT (alternate minimum tax).

WORKING WITH YOUR TAX ADVISER

Do you need a tax adviser? Many of the best prepared tax returns, from the standpoint of accuracy and tax minimization, are prepared by the individual taxpayer. Many people don't mind doing their own taxes if they have the time to become informed about tax-saving matters. If your individual tax situation isn't too complicated, there's nothing wrong with doing your own taxes. It will also save you some money that you, in turn, can save.

On the other hand, for many busy medical professionals, tax preparation and planning is intimidating, frustrating, and generally unpleasant. The extensive tax reforms of the 1980s have managed to confuse just about everybody, and as soon as you begin to feel that you understand the current rules, Congress is probably going to change them. A good tax adviser can be a lifesaver. He or she will help you minimize your tax bill by keeping you informed of strategies you can use and by knowing how different expenses and income are treated. A good tax adviser will help you stay up-to-date on tax-saving techniques and the latest changes in the tax laws.

But you have to work with your tax adviser, because *only you are fully aware of your financial situation*. You shouldn't expect your tax adviser to be a miracle worker who can make sense out of an unorganized mass of receipts and forms you give him or her around April 1st. You should organize your records, keep them organized throughout the year, and always keep tax considerations in mind before making any financial transaction. Simplify your tax life and your tax adviser's job as much as you reasonably can. Consolidate investments, keep the best and most complete records you can, and *avoid all sorts of supposed tax shelters*. Keep a notebook handy to record miscellaneous deductible expenses. Remember, tax minimization and tax planning is a year-round process, so expect your adviser to advise you throughout the year, and listen to the advice. A good tax adviser will be available year-round, not only to answer your questions but also to review the tax implications of contemplated investments and suggest tax-saving strategies.

Whether you prepare your taxes yourself or have a tax adviser, you will benefit from obtaining IRS publications that pertain to your situation. Check the accompanying list of IRS publications. An Income Tax Return Summary work sheet is also provided to help you monitor your year-to-year income and tax trends.

TABLE 5

IRS Publications

These publications, which are available free from the IRS, can be very helpful in understanding income tax matters that pertain to you.

Publication Number	Title
1	Your Rights as a Taxpayer
15	Circular E, Employer's Tax Guide
17	Your Federal Income Tax
54	Tax Guide for U.S. Citizens and Resident Aliens Abroad
334	Tax Guide for Small Business
448	Federal Estate and Gift Taxes
463	Travel, Entertainment, and Gift Expenses
501	Exemptions, Standard Deduction, and Filing Information
502	Medical and Dental Expenses
503	Child and Dependent Care Credit
504	Tax Information for Divorced or Separated Individuals
505	Tax Withholding and Estimated Tax
508	Educational Expenses
510	Excise Taxes
514	Foreign Tax Credit for Individuals

Publication Number	Title
516	Tax Information for U.S. Government Civilian Employees Stationed Abroad
520	Scholarships and Fellowships
521	Moving Expenses
523	Tax Information on Selling Your Home
524	Credit for the Elderly or the Disabled
525	Taxable and Nontaxable Income
526	Charitable Contributions
527	Residential Rental Property
529	Miscellaneous Deductions
530	Tax Information for Homeowners (including Owners of Condominiums and Cooperative Apartments)
533	Self-Employment Tax
534	Depreciation
535	Business Expenses
536	Net Operating Losses
537	Installment Sales
538	Accounting Periods and Methods
541	Tax Information on Partnerships
542	Tax Information on Corporations
544	Sales and Other Dispositions of Assets
545	Interest Expense
547	Nonbusiness Disasters, Casualties, and Thefts
549	Condemnations and Business Casualties and Thefts
550	Investment Income and Expenses
551	Basis of Assets
554	Tax Information for Older Americans
555	Community Property and the Federal Income Tax
556	Examination of Returns, Appeal Rights, and Claims for Refund
559	Tax Information for Survivors, Executors, and Administrators
560	Self-Employed Retirement Plans
561	Determining the Value of Donated Property
564	Mutual Fund Distributions

Publication Number	Title
570	Tax Guide for Individuals in U.S. Possessions
575	Pension and Annuity Income
584	Nonbusiness Disaster, Casualty, and Theft Loss Workbook
586A	The Collection Process (Income Tax Accounts)
587	Business of Your Home
589	Tax Information on S Corporations
590	Individual Retirement Accounts (IRAs)
593	Tax Highlights for U.S. Citizens and Residents Going Abroad
594	The Collection Process (Employment Tax Accounts)
596	Earned Income Credit
901	U.S. Tax Treaties
904	Interrelated Computations for Estate and Gift Taxes
907	Tax Information for Handicapped and Disabled Individuals
908	Bankruptcy and Other Debt Cancellation
909	Alternative Minimum Tax for Individuals
910	Guide to Free Tax Services
911	Tax Information for Direct Sellers
915	Social Security Benefits and Equivalent Railroad Retirement Benefits
916	Information Returns
917	Business Use of a Car
919	Is My Withholding Correct?
925	Passive Activity and At-Risk Rules
926	Employment Taxes for Household Employers
927	Tax Obligations of Legalized Aliens
929	Tax Rules for Children and Dependents
936	Limits on Home Mortgage Interest Deduction
937	Business Reporting
1004	Identification Numbers Under ERISA
1048	Filing Requirements for Employee Benefit Plans
1251	Employee Benefit Plans: Sources of Information

MASTERING THE TAX GAME

Tax planning isn't just a year-round issue: It's a multiyear issue. Sound tax-saving techniques usually take years of planning and often take years to develop fully. One of the best things about multiyear tax planning is that you eventually learn to avoid making mistakes that you have made in the past. Investing in anything for purely tax-driven motives is a mistake. Letting tax

---

INCOME TAX RETURN SUMMARY

This work sheet can be used to record key numbers from your past tax returns. This is a convenient means of monitoring your year-to-year changes in income, deductions, and income tax burden.

	Year					
	.....	.....	.....	.....	.....	.....
Income:						
Wages	$.....	$.....	$.....	$.....	$.....	$.....
Interest	.....	.....	.....	.....	.....	.....
Dividends	.....	.....	.....	.....	.....	.....
Personal business	.....	.....	.....	.....	.....	.....
Capital gains	.....	.....	.....	.....	.....	.....
Pensions	.....	.....	.....	.....	.....	.....
Rents, royalties, partnerships, and trusts	.....	.....	.....	.....	.....	.....
Other	—	—	—	—	—	—
Total income	.....	.....	.....	.....	.....	.....

Note: The following items are not additive; simply indicate the amounts from the appropriate lines on your federal, and in the case of the last line, on your state/local income tax returns:

Total adjustments to income	.....	.....	.....	.....	.....	.....
Total itemized deductions	.....	.....	.....	.....	.....	.....
Taxable income	.....	.....	.....	.....	.....	.....
Federal income tax	.....	.....	.....	.....	.....	.....
State/local income tax	.....	.....	.....	.....	.....	.....

savings get in the way of sound investing and personal financial planning is a mistake.

Many higher income medical professionals have been saddled with soured limited partnership investments. In the worst of instances, they have to continue making installment payments on deals that are failing or have failed. If you are concerned about the status of these investments, you generally don't have any palatable alternatives. While you may be able to sell your partnership investment on a secondary market, good prices are available only on the quality of partnership that you would want to hold on to. Also, there might be adverse income tax consequences if the partnership is sold. Not a very rosy situation, but at the very least, it will be a learning experience. I would like to think that most people will not repeat these mistakes, but alas, some investors spend their lives going from one bad tax-motivated investment to the next. Don't let it be you.

It doesn't take a big time commitment to become "tax aware," it just takes commitment, and you're sure to benefit. Remember that tax aware doesn't mean "tax driven." The days of tax-motivated transactions have, mercifully, come to an end. In spite of an incredibly complex "Infernal" Revenue Code, we are better off, at least to the extent that you are better off by making investment decisions primarily on the basis of their economic merits, and while you need to be aware of the tax implications of your day-to-day personal and business activities, they should no longer be motivated by their impact on your personal tax status.

YEAR-END TAX-SAVING TECHNIQUES

By now you should realize that tax planning is a long term and ongoing process. However, sometimes things just don't work out the way you've planned them, or you realize it's already November and you haven't started to plan them at all. There are a few tricks you can use at the last minute to help cut your current year's tax bill and start planning the next year in advance. These last-minute efforts cannot take the place of sustained, long-term planning.

■ Try to determine whether or not you will be subject to the AMT, either in the current year or the next. In general, you try to accelerate deductions into the current year and defer income to the next year, but AMT provisions disallow certain itemized deductions and may tax income at a higher rate than it would otherwise be subject to. AMT liability must be considered before implementing any tax-saving strategies. Itemized deductions that are treated as exclusion items for AMT purposes should be shifted to years in which you will not be subject to AMT. These include personal interest, state and local taxes, and most miscellaneous itemized deductions. If you are subject to AMT in the current year but will not be in the next, the acceleration of income could result in tax savings, depending on the nature of the AMT preferences or adjustments.

■ Since miscellaneous expenses are deductible only to the extent that they exceed 2 percent of your adjusted gross income, you should tally them up prior to the year's end to see how close you are to the 2-percent hurdle. Miscellaneous expenses include professional dues, tax-preparation fees, unreimbursed employee business expenses, and certain educational costs. To the extent permitted by the regulations, you can either bunch more miscellaneous expenses into the current year or defer them into the next, depending on where you stand. Similarly, you may want to check on whether your taxable income is nearing the 31 percent bracket. If so, you should consider deferring income, to the extent permissible.

■ Medical expenses above 7.5 percent of adjusted gross income are deductible. Just as with miscellaneous expenses, try to bunch them up. If you're close to exceeding 7.5 percent for one year, pay any outstanding bills and prepay any medical procedures that you will be having the next year. If you aren't going to come close to the 7.5 percent floor, on the other hand, put off as many of these expenses as possible, because maybe the next year your medical expenses will be higher. (Let's hope not.)

■ To a certain extent, you can also control when you receive investment income. One way to defer investment income is to transfer funds from instruments that pay current interest, such as money market funds, into Treasury bills or certificates of deposit that mature within a year or less and that won't pay interest until next year. You also have control of when you realize capital gains and losses on stocks and real estate. You may want to consider realizing capital losses to offset any capital gains in a specific year. In addition, you can use net capital losses in excess of capital gains to offset up to $3,000 of other income on a dollar-for-dollar basis. If you plan to make a large charitable contribution in a year in which you intend to recognize a capital gain in securities, you'll get a double tax benefit by making the gift with the securities, although you may need to consider alternative minimum tax (AMT) consequences. Generally, you get a deduction for the full value of the securities you donate, and you won't owe tax on their appreciation.

Postponing income isn't always a great idea, however. If you expect to be in a higher tax bracket next year, then you would try to do the opposite—to accelerate earnings into the current year. In order to decide when to receive the income, you generally have to have a pretty good picture of your tax situation for this year and next.

■ If you have any net income from self-employment, you can open up a Keogh account and tuck away up to 20 percent of those earnings tax free. Many people mistakenly assume that they can't have a Keogh plan for their moonlighting income if they participate in an employer-sponsored pension plan. Although you can contribute to your Keogh plan up to the time you file your tax return, the plan itself must be set up by December 31. An alternative to the Keogh is the Simplified Employee Pension plan, which is more limited in the amount that can be contributed, but which can be set up and funded as late as April 15 of the following year. See Chapter 7 for more details on tax-deferred retirement plans.

■ If you make estimated state income tax payments, rather than paying the last installment in January, you may want to pay it in late December so that it can be deducted this year. Make sure your tax deduction will exceed the amount of interest lost by paying early, however. Also, this strategy won't work if you are subject to the AMT this year.

■ The end of the year 'tis the season to give vent to your charitable impulses. Don't forget that donations of such tangibles as old clothing, furniture, and books are deductible at fair market value. Keep track of any expenses you incur driving your famous chocolate royale pound cake to the church bake sale—your mileage is deductible at twelve cents per mile. Donations of appreciated stock are often even better than cash, since in addition to your income-tax deduction you can avoid paying tax on the capital gain.

■ When you borrow money to invest, any interest you pay on the loan is deductible, but only against investment-related income. If you paid investment interest this year, try to produce enough

They say the only things that are certain in life are death and taxes, but at least death doesn't get worse every time Congress convenes.

investment income to offset it. Capital gains count as investment income for this purpose. Talk to your securities broker about bond (or stock) swaps. You may be able to realize a capital loss by selling a security in which you have a loss and then buying a similar one. You must be careful not to buy the same instrument, which could subject you to the wash sale rules.

■ Set up separate bank accounts for business, personal, investment, and real estate activities. Interest deductibility depends on your activity. If you use just one bank account, it's hard to tell where the money came from and where it went.

■ Make sure your withheld and estimated taxes will equal or exceed either last year's tax bill or 90 percent of what you'll owe for the current year. If you think you'll come up short, there may still be time to compensate by increasing your withholding for the rest of the year.

The income tax action plan will help remind you of important aspects to keep in mind as you go through this year-round process.

INCOME TAX ACTION PLAN

Current Status		
Needs Action	Okay or Not Applicable	
☐	☐	1. Familiarize yourself with the tax advantages available to medical professionals.
☐	☐	2. Carefully analyze any investment or transaction that is being recommended to you or that you intend to make primarily on the basis of tax saving.
☐	☐	3. Coordinate your income tax planning with other important personal financial-planning areas, including investments and retirement planning.

Current Status		
Needs Action	Okay or Not Applicable	
☐	☐	4. If you are considering establishing or buying a practice, be sure to discuss with a qualified accountant or lawyer how the business should be structured.
☐	☐	5. If you own or are a partner in a practice, become familiar with the tax advantages available to self-employed professionals.
☐	☐	6. Don't lose sight of the role of "old-fashioned" tax-advantaged investments, such as tax-exempt bonds and buying and holding stock and real estate.
☐	☐	7. If you, like many medical professionals, may be subject to the AMT, you should incorporate AMT considerations in your tax planning.
☐	☐	8. Maintain complete and well-organized income tax records throughout the year. Your tax record keeping should be coordinated with your personal record-keeping system.
☐	☐	9. Effective income tax planning is both a year-round process and a multiyear process. Spend some time after tax season with your adviser, if applicable, planning your income tax strategies over the next five years.

Comments:_____

_____

_____

_____

_____

_____

Tax Planning "To Do" List:_____

_____

_____

_____

_____

_____

III

PLANNING FOR LATER LIFE

—

7

Retiring in Good Wealth as Well as Good Health

RETIREMENT REALITIES

All of the financial planning you do during your working years, from investing wisely to insuring against the unforeseen, helps you on your way to your ultimate financial goal—achieving financial security by the time you retire. Yet, retirement planning per se is all too often neglected. Even for higher income people, a secure retirement requires a lifetime of planning. Sadly, many medical professionals overlook the importance of providing for retirement and end up working beyond their desired retirement age and/or enduring a less than financially comfortable retirement.

People who work in the health-care industry often have to plan particularly carefully to assure a financially secure retirement for several reasons.

■ Because of the long duration of education and training, medical careers are shorter than other careers.
■ Many persons in the health-care business are self-employed, and, therefore, they must take the initiative to establish and maintain their own retirement plans.
■ Health-care professionals are, as a group, quite affluent. In order to maintain an affluent life-style during retirement, considerable savings and investments must be amassed.

■ Like other professionals, medical professionals are often too busy during their working years to pay adequate attention to retirement planning. They may simply slough off the need to plan for old age, saying, in effect, "I'm making a lot of money now and putting some of it away. Of course I'll be able to afford to retire." Unfortunately, some may have a rude awakening, either when they retire or a few years into retirement.

There are several other elements that affect the retirement planning process for all of us and may well influence the way you plan for your own retirement.

■ Working people in increasing numbers have set very ambitious retirement expectations. First, and for the first time, most of us expect to retire with no diminution in life-style. Previous generations expected to cut back when they retired—not any longer. Second, many people aspire to retire early. More and more people are realizing the dream of early retirement, although many end up (or will end up) regretting it.

■ Life expectancy has increased dramatically since the beginning of this century. The notion of letting people retire at age 65 was advanced at a time when few working people attained that age. Now, a person who reaches 65 should plan on living another twenty-five years, and many will live well beyond age 90. This requires a lot of money. A doctor or dentist may work for thirty-five years, during which he or she will have to accumulate a retirement fund that is large enough to last twenty-five years or more.

■ Higher inflation (compared to what was experienced prior to the 1970s) seems to be firmly entrenched in our economy. High inflation makes it tougher to accumulate resources in advance of retirement and makes it tougher to maintain an adequate living standard throughout a long retirement.

■ Fiscal pressures on the government and employers mean that working people will have to rely less on Social Security and company pension plans and rely more on personal savings and investments to assure an adequate retirement income.

Retirement planning is like good health care. The earlier you start treatment, the less it hurts later.

IT'S NEVER TOO EARLY OR TOO LATE TO START PLANNING FOR RETIREMENT

Don't despair over your retirement prospects. You are fortunate to be working in a profession that, for the most part, offers job security and above-average—if not high—earning potential. However, the earlier you begin planning for retirement, the better. The following example shows just how dramatic the delay in setting aside money for retirement can be.

Example: If a 30-year-old saves 10 percent of his or her gross income every year until age 65, the income from that nest egg alone, combined with Social Security, will provide a very comfortable retirement. Pension income, if any, is icing on the cake. If someone waits until age 40 to begin, they have to save between 20 and 25 percent of their income over the next 25 years in order to retire comfortably on nest egg and Social Security alone. If this person waits until age 50 and has no pension benefits, the amount he or she will have to save jumps to over 50 percent of gross income per year! Since Uncle Sam takes out at least another 25 percent, the 50-year-old would have to live on only one-quarter of his or her income for 15 years in order to accumulate the funds necessary to provide a comfortable retirement. Can't be done.

So the time to start planning for retirement is now. This chapter will show you how to:

1. Estimate how much income you will need during retirement;
2. Figure out how much you will need to accumulate in order to fund a comfortable retirement;
3. Take stock of your progress in meeting your retirement needs;
4. Take action to suture the gap between the resources you now have and the resources you will eventually need to retire.

You can use the checklists and work sheets provided to help you get on the right track.

You really don't need to begin saving for retirement before you reach age 60. At that point, simply save 250 percent of your income each year, and you'll be able to retire comfortably at age 70.

A PRELIMINARY EXAMINATION OF YOUR RETIREMENT PLANNING STATUS

1. ESTIMATE HOW MUCH INCOME YOU WILL NEED DURING RETIREMENT

If you are many years from retirement, estimating your income requirements at retirement age may be of little concern to you now, but you should at least pay some attention to your retirement aspirations. After all, you may well spend almost one-third of your life retired. If, on the other hand, you are nearing retirement age, you must begin to think about your retirement life-style, including the all-important decision about where you want to live.

Once you have an idea of how you want to live in retirement, you can estimate your expenses, first in current dollars and then in future, inflated dollars. In order to maintain the same standard of living in retirement that you enjoyed during your working years, you will need annual retirement income of approximately 75 percent of the amount you *spend* per year during your working years.

> *Example:* The Garners are going to retire in a few months. Last year, they had total income of $145,000, but they saved about $25,000 of that, including a contribution to Dr. Garner's retirement plan. Based upon the 75 percent rule of thumb, they will need about $90,000 in their first year of retirement to maintain an equivalent standard of living. The calculation is as follows: Since they saved $25,000 of their $145,000 income, they *spent* $120,000; 75 percent of $120,000 is $90,000.

Depending upon your circumstances and desires, you may need more or less than 75 percent of your pre-retirement income. If you are under 50, make some well-thought-out approximations of what your expenses would be if you were to retire today. If you are within ten to fifteen years of retirement, you should put pencil to paper to prepare a detailed retirement living expense budget. As best you can, try to quantify your retirement expenses. Think about how you expect your life-style to change. You will find that some costs decline, including work-related expenses and income taxes (but not dramatically). Social Security withholding taxes drop to zero unless you work part-time. Other costs will increase, including health care (be sure to provide for health insurance), and if you are so inclined, travel. Many people decide they would like to try alternative housing arrangements—living in a condominium rather than a single family house, for example. Ideally, any major changes should be undertaken, or at least experienced before—not during—retirement. During retirement, when funds are limited, you don't want to realize that a life-style change was not at all what you wanted.

One of the biggest mistakes that people make in planning for their retirement is either ignoring or underestimating the effects of inflation. Even though inflation is much lower now than it was during the double-digit days of 1979–1981, it still takes its toll on your purchasing power. Many retirees, in particular, see their purchasing power diminished by inflation, since much of their income is either fixed (like many retirement annuities) or lags inflation somewhat (like Social Security). So when you project your retirement expenses, you must first consider inflation from now until you retire, and then you must factor in inflation for all of your retirement years. Now, you might ask, what rate of inflation should one assume? This is a crucial question. If you were retiring around 1970 and you looked at the inflation rate over the 1950 to 1970 period, you may well have guessed that inflation would continue as it had—at around 2 percent per annum! Projecting inflation is a tricky business, but it must be done. Many experts now recommend that people who are making financial projections assume a future annual rate of inflation of 4 to 5 percent. Some experts think that even higher inflation rates are in the offing. Incidentally, the average annual inflation rate during the 1980s, including the high rates of the early 1980s, was 4.7 percent. I use a rate of 4.5 percent when I make my projections. As the following example shows, inflation can take a heavy toll on purchasing power.

Example: Dr. and Mrs. McCardle turned 50 this year, and are now hard at work trying to figure out how much income they will need in order to be able to afford to retire at age 65. They now figure that in order to live like they want to when they retire, they will need $65,000 of income from pensions and personal investments per year (including taxes) in addition to Social Security. Of course, $65,000 would suffice if they were to retire today, but they will need more than that fifteen years hence to have the same purchasing power as $65,000 of income today. In fact, at an assumed inflation rate of 4.5 percent, they will need over $125,000 of income at age 65 in order to enjoy the same life-style that $65,000 fetches today.

2. FIGURE OUT HOW MUCH YOU WILL NEED TO ACCUMULATE IN ORDER TO FUND A COMFORTABLE RETIREMENT

Once you have estimated how much you expect to spend when you retire, you need to forecast how much you will need to accumulate personally in addition to estimated Social Security and pension benefits to provide for your needs for the rest of your life. The so-called "three legs of the retirement stool" are pension, Social Security, and personal resources. Job related income can reduce Social Security benefits. Before making the actual calculations, two important matters must be considered—life expectancy and inflation during your retirement years. Retirees are living, hopefully happily, for many years. But many who retired quite comfortably twenty or so years ago are struggling financially. They simply weren't prepared to fund so many years of retirement during a period of high inflation. So life expectancy and inflation *must* be considered. Whether the thought appeals to you or not, you should plan on living until at least age 90. (The current joint and last-survivor life expectancy of a couple who are both age 50 is thirty-nine years!) So if you are going to retire at age 65, you will need enough resources to tide you over for at least twenty-five years. By the way, I'm a strong advocate of spending it all before you and your spouse die, but please don't plan to spend it all before you reach 90.

Inflation exacts a heavy toll on retirees, particularly those whose income consists mainly of fixed annuities and Social Security. We should return to the McCardles, who are preparing retirement projections:

> *Example:* In the previous example, the somewhat startled McCardles found out they were going to need an income of $125,000 when they retire at 65, fifteen years hence, to have the same purchasing power that $65,000 has today. As if this isn't bad enough, things get worse. Inflation doesn't go away when you retire. When the McCardles reach age 75, they will need just shy of $200,000 (at a 4.5-percent inflation rate) to have the purchasing power that $65,000 had twenty-five years earlier. Of course, inflation may end up being less than 4.5 percent, but it could be more. Inflation affects many retirees *somewhat* less than it does working people, since housing and fuel costs, which are often reduced in retirement, are major contributors to the inflation rate.

3. EVALUATE YOUR PROGRESS IN MEETING YOUR RETIREMENT NEEDS

Estimating how much you will need to accumulate by the time you reach retirement age can be startling. If you are still young, this amount may seem more like the gross national product of a small country, but it is probably attainable without enduring a lot of deprivation. At this point you need to tally up the assets you already have available that will eventually be used for retirement purposes. All your savings—except those that are earmarked for specific nonretirement-related purposes, such as savings for the down payment on a home or savings for educating the kids—will eventually be available to support you during retirement. If you completed the Personal Balance Sheet in Chapter 1, you have already summarized the value of your investments. Two caveats: Don't include the value of your home in your retirement-related assets, unless you plan to sell the house and become a renter when you retire. Don't include the value of your personal property, because it isn't worth anything to anyone else anyway—unless you have collectibles, which in many instances still don't fetch very much.

As you review your current retirement planning status, there is one other matter that you should consider—housing costs. If you can be mortgage free or have a very low mortgage by the time you retire, your living expenses will be considerably lower than if you remain saddled with a large mortgage or if you rent. As part of your retirement planning, you should probably strive to be mortgage free by the time you retire.

4. SUTURE THE GAP BETWEEN THE RESOURCES YOU NOW HAVE AND THE RESOURCES YOU WILL NEED FOR RETIREMENT

If you have taken the pains to figure out how much you need to be able to retire in comfort, you probably realize—if you hadn't already—that you don't yet have enough money in the kitty to meet your needs. You should take heart in the fact that very few people achieve financial independence until they are very near retirement age anyway. What is most important now is to make sure you take the action that is necessary to meet your financial needs *throughout* your retirement. The Retirement Planning Work Sheet allows you to compute the annual savings required in order to accumulate the resources you will need for retirement.

There is no magic behind accumulating the necessary resources for retirement. You can use the investment strategies that were discussed in Chapter 5 to learn how to increase savings and invest wisely. Fortunately, the tax regulations still look favorably upon retirement-earmarked investments. Many of these tax-advantaged plans merit your consideration.

RETIREMENT PLANNING WORK SHEET

Use this three-part work sheet to forecast the amount of retirement income you will require and to estimate the amount of savings you will have to accumulate to meet your retirement income needs.

I. RETIREMENT EXPENSE FORECASTER

This section helps you approximate the amount of annual retirement income that will allow you to maintain your pre-retirement standard of living. First, the approximate income necessary to maintain current living standard in current dollars is calculated. Then, by reference to future value tables and by using the assumed rate of inflation, you can project this amount to your estimated retirement date.

Current gross annual income[1]	$..........
Minus amount of annual savings[2]	(..........)
Subtotal (the amount you spend currently)	....
Multiplied by 75%[3]	x .75
Equals approximate annual cost (in current dollars) of maintaining your current standard of living, if you were retiring this year	$..........
Multiplied by inflation factor (Refer to Inflation Factor Table below)[4]	x....
Equals approximate annual cost (in future dollars) of maintaining your current standard of living when you retire	$..........

INFLATION FACTOR TABLE

Number of Years until Retirement	Factor
5	1.2
10	1.6
15	1.9
20	2.4
25	3.0
30	3.7
35	4.7
40	5.8

Notes:
1. "Current gross annual income" includes all income from all sources.
2. "Annual savings" includes, in addition to the usual sources of savings, reinvested dividends and capital gains, and any contributions to retirement plans that are taken from your annual income.

3. The 75% multiplier is a general rule of thumb that says, in essence, that a retiree can maintain his/her pre-retirement standard of living by spending roughly 75 percent of his/her pre-retirement income. Of course, individual circumstances may dictate a higher or lower percentage. Ideally, you should prepare a retirement budget that details expected expenses. You may find a multiplier less than 75 percent in some circumstances (for example, low housing costs due to paid-off mortgage) or, in other circumstances, a higher multiplier (for example, extensive travel plans).

4. In order to project retirement expenses to retirement age, current-dollar living expenses must be multiplied by a factor to account for inflationary increases. The inflation Factor table can be used for that purpose. The assumed long-term inflation rate is 4.5 percent.

II. RETIREMENT RESOURCES FORECASTER

This section can be used to forecast pension and Social Security benefits at retirement age and then to approximate the aggregate amount of savings/investments that will be needed by retirement age to cover any shortfall between Social Security/pension benefits and your total income needs.

	Current Dollars	Times Inflation Factor[1]	Future (Retirement Age) Dollars
1. Estimated annual living expenses at retirement age (from Part I)			$..........
2. Annual pension income (projection at retirement age available from employer)[2]	$...... x	.... =	....
3. Plus annual Social Security benefits (projection at retirement age available from Social Security Administration)[3]	$...... x	.... =	....
4. Subtotal projected pension and Social Security income (add Lines 2 and 3)			....
5. Shortfall (if expenses are greater than income) that must be funded out of personal savings/investments (subtract Line 4 from Line 1)			....
6. Multiplied by 17[4]			.....x 17
7. Equals amount of savings/investments in future dollars that need to be accumulated by retirement age to fund retirement[5]			$..........

Notes:
1. Use Inflation Factor Table for the appropriate calculation.
2. Employers usually provide pension plan projections at retirement age, expressed in current dollars. If so, the amount should be multiplied by an inflation factor to approximate benefits in future dollars.

3. Social Security estimates are expressed in current dollars and therefore they should be adjusted for inflation similar to note 2 above.

4. As a general rule of thumb, for every $1,000 of annual income you will need to fund at retirement age, you will need to have at least $17,000 in savings/investments in order to keep up with inflation. If you plan to retire before age 62, use a factor of 20, rather than 17.

5. You may be dismayed by the magnitude of the amount of personal resources that you will need to fund your retirement, which can easily exceed $1 million for younger persons and/or people with minimal pension benefits. Nevertheless, good savings habits combined with the power of compounding can usually close the gap between current resources and eventual needs.

III. RETIREMENT SAVINGS ESTIMATOR

This section can be used to estimate the annual amount of savings that are required to accumulate the funds necessary to meet your retirement objectives. The amount computed on Line 7 equals the required *first-year* savings. The annual savings should be increased by five percent in each succeeding year until you retire.

1. Amount of savings/investments in future dollars
   that need to be accumulated by retirement age
   to fund retirement (from Part II) $.........
2. Minus resources that are currently available for
   retirement purposes[1] $..........
3. Multiplied by appreciation factor (refer to Annual Appreciation
   Factor Table below)[2]   x ......
4. Equals estimated future value of retirement
   resources that are currently available
   (multiply Line 2 by Line 3)   (.........)
5. Retirement funds needed by retirement age
   (subtract Line 4 from Line 1)   ....
6. Multiplied by annual savings factor (refer to the Annual Savings
   Factor Table below)[3]   x ......
7. Equals savings needed over the next
   year (multiply Line 5 by Line 6)[4] $.........

Annual Appreciation Factor Table		Annual Savings Factor Table	
Number of Years until Retirement	Factor	Number of Years until Retirement	Factor
5	1.4	5	.1513
10	2.1	10	.0558
15	3.0	15	.0274
20	4.2	20	.0151
25	6.1	25	.0088
30	8.8	30	.0054
35	12.6	35	.0034
40	18.0	40	.0022

Notes:

1. Resources that are currently available typically include the current value of all of your investment-related assets that are not expected to be used before retirement. Don't include the value of your home unless you expect to sell it to raise money for retirement. Don't include any vested pension benefits if you have already factored them in on Line 2 of Part II of this work sheet.

2. The appreciation factor is used to estimate what your currently available retirement resources will be worth when you retire. The appreciation factor assumes a 7.5 percent *after-tax* rate of appreciation.

3. The annual savings factor computes the amount you will need to save during the next year in order to begin accumulating the retirement fund needed by retirement age as indicated on Line 5. The annual savings factor assumes a 7.5 percent *after-tax* rate of return.

4. The annual savings needed to accumulate your retirement nest egg assumes that you will increase the amount of money you save by five percent each year until retirement.

TAX-ADVANTAGED RETIREMENT PLANS— PROVEN MEDICINE FOR ACUTE "CAN'T- AFFORD-TO-RETIRE-ITIS"

The following is a brief summary of plans and investment vehicles that are designed to accumulate money for retirement. All of these plans have tax advantages. Some are more advantageous than others, however. The best plans, of course, cost you nothing. These are pension plans where your employer makes the contributions. The second-best plans are where your employer makes partial contributions. Although these plans cost you some money, you should almost without exception participate in them to the maximum. People give me a lot of excuses for why they don't participate in company-subsidized plans, and all of their excuses are lame. Next in line are retirement-oriented plans, where you make *tax-deductible* contributions. Last on the list, but still worthy of your consideration, are plans or investments whose contributions are not tax deductible, but the income from which is *tax deferred* until retirement. In fact, all of the following retirement-oriented plans and investments at least have the advantage of tax deferral.

Keep in mind that there is a quid pro quo to making retirement-oriented investments. Your money is generally going to be tied up at least until you reach age 59½. So you need to make sure that you will have ready access to some money, should the need arise, by keeping some investments, at least, outside of your retirement plans. Some critics will tell you that since tax rates are currently much lower than they used to be, the benefits of tax deferral are not sufficient to offset the disadvantage of illiquidity. My feeling is that liquidity is of secondary importance compared with the need for people to put aside money regularly that is earmarked for retirement. Anyway, the most vocal critics of tax-deferred investing happen to be investment firms and advisers, who are losing business as a result of people wisely placing more of their money in retirement-oriented plans.

EMPLOYER-SPONSORED PLANS

These plans are for the most part either wholly or partially subsidized by your employer.

PENSION PLANS

As mentioned earlier, health-care providers are becoming hard-pressed to fund generous pension plans, and therefore, the burden of accumulating retirement funds is shifting to the indi-

---

Retirement income has always been viewed as a three-legged stool, consisting of your employer's pension plan, Social Security, and personal resources. Unfortunately, employers and Uncle Sam have been sawing off portions of their legs.

vidual. Nevertheless, if you work for an institution that has a pension plan, and you stay with the institution for a long time, you may retire with a pension that goes a long way toward covering your retirement needs. The important thing to do now, however, is to find out through the projections provided by your employer just how generous the plan is. You may also be permitted to make additional after-tax contributions to the plan, although you should be careful not to put too many eggs in one basket, and if you have a high income, your additional contributions may in fact reduce the amount your employer makes on your behalf.

If you ever leave a company in which you have vested pension benefits, by all means roll the benefits over into an individual retirement account (IRA) within the 60-day limit, if the employer pays you your vested portion. Younger people, in particular, are inclined to view a relatively small check as unimportant for their retirement. Many end up doing something stupid with the money, like buying a car. Not only are they heavily taxed and penalized on their profligacy, they also sacrifice some resources that may be important to their retirement well-being. Incidentally, chronic job hoppers, even if they dutifully roll over whatever pension benefits they receive, usually end up with far less pension income than those who are less peripatetic, because most large institution pension plans are skewed heavily in favor of those employees who have many years of service.

EMPLOYEE THRIFT AND SAVINGS PLANS

These plans usually require you to make after-tax contributions, which are either wholly or partially matched by your employer's contributions. Even though there are no immediate tax benefits, you are getting something for nothing (your employer's contribution), and you will benefit from tax deferral.

401(K) PLANS

401(k) plans, also called salary reduction plans, are one of the best inventions since thumbs. These plans rely primarily on voluntary employee contributions, although employers often contribute to them as well. In addition to the benefit of tax deferral on the income from your 401(k) investments, your annual contributions to the plan, which are deducted from your salary, are not reported as income. Therefore, your salary reductions are the equivalent of a tax-deductible contribution. There is, however, an annual cap on these tax-favored contributions, which is adjusted for inflation each year. If your employer has one, 401(k) plans are simply too good to pass up.

You will probably be required to manage your 401(k) plan investments by specifying the allocation of your plan assets among various investment choices, usually some mutual funds and a guaranteed investment (or guaranteed income) contract (GIC). Many 401(k) holders allocate far too much to the GICs. Over the long run, a mix of stock and bond mutual funds will usually provide a superior return. The important thing here, similar to all your investments, is to avoid investing in extremes. Perhaps a split of 50 percent in stock funds and 50 percent in interest-earning funds (including the GIC) will suit you fine. Many investment experts recommend a 50–60 percent exposure to stocks, especially for people under age 50. If, and this is unlikely for health-care professionals but may pertain to your spouse, you have a 401(k) option of investing a portion of your money in the stock of your employer, I would invest only a nominal amount, if any, in "own-company" stock. What you need most in a 401(k) plan is diversification, and chances are that you (or your spouse) already own a lot of this stock through stock purchase plans.

403(B) PLANS

Many health-care professionals work for nonprofit hospitals or other nonprofit organizations. Many such institutions offer 403(b) plans (often called "tax-sheltered annuities"), which are similar to 401(k)s. Your taxable income is reduced by the amount of your contributions, and the earnings on your investments are tax deferred until you begin making withdrawals. Also similar to a 401(k), there are limitations on the amount you can contribute. You can have both a 401(k) plan and a 403(b) plan, but the total contributions to both cannot exceed the 403(b) limitations.

How you invest your 403(b) funds depends upon the options that your employer makes available to you. When you have some choice, such as stock funds or bond funds, follow the same general investment allocation approach that was outlined for 401(k) plan investments.

The only way you can live comfortably on Social Security is if you live only one week of each month.

SELF-EMPLOYED RETIREMENT PLANS

Many health-care professionals are self-employed either full- or part-time, and therefore are eligible to set up their own retirement plan. Moonlighters, even if they are employed by another organization that has a pension plan, can probably still set up a self-employed plan as well. If you have any income from self-employment, you should establish a self-employed retirement plan. There are two categories of plans to consider.

KEOGH PLANS

Keogh plans are specifically structured to allow self-employed people—sole proprietors and partners—to set up their own retirement savings programs. Most Keoghs are set up as defined-contribution plans, and they can be structured to allow you to contribute, and deduct, up to 25 percent of your net income from self-employment (actually 20 percent of your income before you make the contribution) or $30,000, whichever is less. You can tailor the plan to meet your own needs and resources. If, as is often the case with self-employed physicians and dentists, you have employees, you must extend this benefit to them and make contributions at the same percentage-of-income level that you do for yourself. If you have employees, you should weigh the costs of making contributions on behalf of your employees against the benefits you receive.

In some instances a *defined-benefit* Keogh plan may be a wonderful means of accumulating a substantial retirement nest egg. Generally, these plans are appropriate for doctors, dentists, or other high income health-care professionals who are over 50 and who have no employees. A defined-benefit plan can be structured to allow very high annual tax-deductible contributions, well in excess of the $30,000 cap on defined-contribution Keoghs. I've seen these plans work very well for high-income doctors and others who have been remiss in setting up a pension plan in the past and have a lot of catching up to do.

Remember that your Keogh plan must be established by December 31 of the tax year when you want to begin taking the deduction, even though you can delay making the contribution until your tax return is filed—including extensions—in the succeeding year. If you missed the deadline, but it is not yet April 15, you can set up a SEP, which is described below. Some health-care providers never know when to retire. They may continue to make contributions to their Keogh plan after reaching age 70½, as long as they still report self-employment income.

SIMPLIFIED EMPLOYEE PENSION PLANS

As the name suggests, simplified employee pension plans (affectionately known as SEPs, and they're easy to love) are simple to set up, simple to maintain, and simply wonderful retirement savings vehicles for self-employed health-care professionals. Instead of maintaining a separate pension plan as is required with a Keogh, SEP contributions are deposited into your (and if applicable, your employees') IRA account(s). You may establish a SEP after the end of the tax year in which you want to begin taking the deduction as long as it is set up and funded before April 15. Generally, the amount you may contribute is 15 percent of your gross self-employment income, up to $30,000 per annum. You can also kick in an IRA contribution on top of the SEP contribution. As with Keoghs, nondiscrimination rules apply if you have employees. Finally, chronic workers can still contribute to a SEP after age 70½.

INDIVIDUAL RETIREMENT ACCOUNTS

Everyone who has earned income is still eligible to contribute to an IRA and enjoy the benefits of tax deferral. Unfortunately, as you probably know, not everyone can still deduct IRA contributions. Also unfortunately, many people use nondeductibility as an excuse to forgo making any IRA payments. I may be a lone voice in the wilderness, but I think a nondeductible IRA can still play an important role as a retirement savings vehicle. Even though you may already participate in a couple of retirement-oriented plans, it probably isn't enough. So if you need to sock away more retirement money, why not do it through an IRA account, ideally at a good no-load mutual fund company? Then use your IRA money to buy some good quality stock and bond funds, or take the easy way out and buy a balanced fund, which contains both stocks and bonds.

DEFERRED ANNUITIES AND CASH VALUE LIFE INSURANCE

Insurance companies offer a variety of products that have tax-deferred savings features. A deferred annuity is similar to a nondeductible IRA, in that earnings on the money in the annuity accumulate, tax deferred, until withdrawal. Deferred annuities are no different from any other insurance product in that the details of the annuity contract, including fees and commissions, are almost impossible to understand. Choosing the right one for your specific needs can be very difficult. Unfortunately, while there are dramatic differences among annuities in terms of fees, rates of return, and flexibility, few people go to the effort to search for the right one. Instead, like most insurance products, they are usually sold, not bought. You might want to consider investing in a deferred annuity as part of your retirement savings program, but—because of the complexity and costs associated with them—only after you have taken full advantage of the other tax-advantaged retirement plans described above.

Cash value life insurance comes in many forms, including single premium, universal, and variable. While these policies afford some life insurance protection, they are often used to accumulate tax-deferred savings for retirement. But the cash value of these policies grows slowly during the initial years of ownership, because much of your premium is used to cover commissions and administrative costs. Even over the long term, the costs that go into maintaining these policies can drag down returns. Therefore, similar to deferred annuities, you can often get more bang for your buck by investing in other retirement-oriented savings plans.

OTHER MATTERS THAT MANY NEED ATTENTION

EXCESS DISTRIBUTIONS

The 1986 "Tax Complification" Act imposes a 15 percent tax on so-called "excess distributions" from qualified retirement plans, IRAs, and 403(b) annuity contracts. Like most of the provisions of the act, the rules are very complicated. Suffice it to say that if you are fortunate enough to expect an annual income from your retirement plan(s) in excess of $150,000 or you expect to take a lump-sum distribution in excess of $750,000, you should speak with an income-tax professional about your potential exposure to this onerous tax. The threshold amounts are indexed for inflation, so if you are many years from retirement, you may escape being subject to this tax. It all depends upon how much you will have accumulated.

CHOOSING BETWEEN A LUMP SUM AND AN ANNUITY

While some pension plans require you to take an annuity when you retire, your plan may allow you the option of taking a lump-sum payout. There may be some advantage to taking a lump sum, but this option must be considered carefully.

If the monthly payments provided by an annuity are not adjusted for inflation (most are not), and if you are confident that you or your investment adviser can invest the lump-sum amount more profitably, then the lump-sum option may be a good choice, if it is available. You'll probably be able to generate more income than the annuity and at the same time cope better with inflation. There may be a serious drawback to taking a lump sum, however. If you or your spouse should incur substantial uninsured medical expenses, such as a long-term hospital or nursing home stay, or should otherwise be subject to the claims of creditors or the mismanagement of money that may occur in old age, your lump-sum retirement fund may be jeopardized. In the worst instances, this could seriously erode or altogether wipe out your pension resources. This eventuality must be weighed carefully in deciding on the lump-sum option as opposed to an annuity. Money that is in an annuity is usually protected from these adverse occurrences. What is the solution? As we have said, nothing in personal financial planning is either/or. Perhaps a partial lump-sum settlement and partial annuity may be a desirable compromise. If you opt for an annuity, don't necessarily take the first one that's offered to you. Payout rates on so-called "immediate-pay" annuities vary widely. Shop around for the company that offers the most attractive terms. If you take a lump sum, you have some homework to do as well. You may be able to take advantage of forward averaging to reduce the tax impact of the distribution, or if you can afford it, you can further postpone taxes on the plan distribution by rolling it over into an IRA. This way, you won't pay tax until you begin withdrawing money from the IRA.

Live it up when you're retired. Spend your kids' inheritance. Spread the word (to everyone but my parents!).

MANAGING YOUR RETIREMENT PLAN
INVESTMENTS

Depending on your situation, you probably are responsible for managing part, if not most or all, of your retirement plan investments. First, you should summarize *all* of your investments periodically—your retirement plan investments and your personal investments. The reason for this is quite simple—you cannot make investment decisions intelligently without knowing the status of all of your investments. The Investment Allocation Analysis work sheet in Chapter 5 will assist you in summarizing your total investment situation. The approach to managing retirement-earmarked investments really isn't any different from managing your other investments. The following suggestions may be helpful for managing your investments prudently.

■ Never invest in extremes. As explained in Chapters 4 and 5, your total investment portfolio should consist of appropriate portions of stock, interest-earning, and perhaps, real estate investments. If you find that most of your investments are concentrated in a single investment category, you are probably either taking too much or too little risk.

■ As you near retirement age, perhaps within ten years of retirement, you should gradually begin to increase the proportion of your total investment portfolio (not just retirement funds) that is invested in more conservative, interest-earning investments. The reason for this is that you have less time to make up for a downturn in the stock market, which, as we all know, happens from time to time. You still need exposure to stocks, however, and this exposure will continue well into your retirement years. Why? As we saw earlier in this chapter, inflation doesn't go away when you retire, and you therefore need the inflation hedge that stocks have provided, and hopefully, will continue to provide.

■ You can minimize current income taxes somewhat by loading up your retirement plan investments with highly taxed securities and concentrating your personal investments in tax-advantaged securities.

Example: Dr. Toothman, a dentist, has $1,000,000 in investments—half in her Simplified Employee Pension (SEP) plan and half in her personal portfolio. She likes to buy and hold stocks, she likes U.S. savings bonds, and she likes both stock and corporate bond mutual funds. Rather than mix up these investments among her SEP plan and her personal portfolio, she should load up the SEP with stock and bond mutual funds and emphasize individually purchased stocks and savings bonds in her personal portfolio. This strategy will minimize the income taxes she will have to pay on her investment income. Although stock and corporate bond mutual funds are highly taxed investments, since they pass on dividend and interest income and realized capital gains to the investor, this income will not be taxed as long as these investments are in her SEP. On the other hand, individually owned stocks are tax-advantaged insofar as no capital gains are paid until they are sold. Since she likes to buy and hold, she can benefit from keeping these in her personal portfolio and letting them appreciate in value without paying any taxes. Similarly, interest on U.S. savings bonds can accumulate tax free until they mature, so she is quite correct to keep them in her personal portfolio.

EARLY RETIREMENT

Ahhh, early retirement. How many times have you dreamed of early retirement over the past week? Many health-care professionals, because they work hard and are generally well paid, look forward to being able to retire early. If you are one of them, you have your financial work cut out for you. Early retirees face a potential double whammy: they have fewer years to accumulate sufficient resources to fund a longer period of retirement. Personal savings and investments play an even more important role for the early retiree. A couple of rules of thumb to keep in mind: If you would have to rely on your retirement accounts and/or Social Security benefits to meet living expenses before age 65, you may not be able to afford an early retirement. If a significant amount of your retirement income is going to be fixed—in the form of an annuity, for example—and once you are retired you will not be able to save a generous portion of it to help fund increased future living costs, you may not be able to afford an early retirement.

The above caveats notwithstanding, it is possible to retire early and comfortably. But you need to plan for it far in advance. Physicians, dentists, and other health-care professionals can often take a somewhat different approach to early retirement. Many have the option of gradually reducing their working schedule, which, in many respects, is the best solution of all. First, you get a taste of retirement without summarily leaving the working world (some people actually don't enjoy not working). Second, you still have some income coming in. Third, you can get an idea of how it feels to live on a reduced income.

After reading this chapter, you may think that you won't be able to retire until you're 95. But remember, virtually everything you do to improve and preserve your financial well-being during your working life is helping you prepare for retirement. Many people get a late start on saving for retirement and yet they manage quite well. All of the financial hurdles you have or will have to conquer, like paying off education loans, starting your practice, buying a home, and educating the children, have been preparing you for the sacrifices that may be necessary to fund a comfortable retirement. You've succeeded in the past, and you will succeed in your retirement planning. The following Retirement Planning Timetable and Retirement Action Plan will help guide you.

RETIREMENT PLANNING TIMETABLE

It's never too early to plan for retirement. To prepare for a financially comfortable retirement, you need to take action throughout your working years. The following timetable describes important steps to take at various ages to help you on your way.

Retirement Planning Timetable

It's never too early to plan for retirement. To prepare for a financially comfortable retirement, you need to take action throughout your working years. The following timetable describes important steps to take at various ages to help you on your way.

DURING ALL WORKING YEARS

1. Make sure you always have adequate and continuous insurance coverage.
2. Consider the ramifications on future pension benefits of any contemplated job change. Job-hopping can curtail pension benefits severely.
3. Roll over any vested pension benefits you receive as a result of a job change into an IRA or other tax-deferred retirement plan.

BEFORE AGE 40

1. Contribute regularly to an IRA or other retirement-earmarked savings fund.
2. Purchase a home so that by the time you retire your housing costs will be under control.
3. Discuss the fine points of the pension plan with your company's benefits officer.

AGES 40–49

1. Periodically check with Social Security by requesting and filing Form SSA-7004. You will receive a "Personal Earnings and Benefit Estimate Statement" to verify that your wages are being properly credited to your account and to prepare your retirement income projections.
2. Analyze personal assets, and work out a plan for funding an adequate retirement income.
3. Actively manage your IRA and other retirement funds with appropriate emphasis on capital-gains-oriented investments.
4. Make a will, and review it every three years or when moving to another state. Discuss other estate planning techniques with an experienced estate planning attorney.

AGES 50–59

1. Continue to request your Social Security "Personal Earnings and Benefit Estimate Statement" periodically.
2. Review your status with your company's pension plan regularly.
3. Revise your retirement income and expense projections, taking inflation into consideration.
4. Confirm the beneficiary designations on life insurance policies.
5. Start gradually shifting some of your IRA and other retirement-earmarked funds into lower risk investments with more emphasis on yield.
6. Join the American Association of Retired Persons to take advantage of the many sources of information and help that they offer. The address is:

   AARP
   1909 K Street, N.W.
   Washington D.C. 20049

AGES 60–64

1. If you are contemplating an early retirement, discuss the advantages and disadvantages with your employer's personnel officer and the local Social Security office.
2. Collect the documents necessary to process Social Security benefits:
   - Both spouses' Social Security cards
   - Proof of both spouses' ages
   - Marriage certificate
   - Copy of latest income tax withholding statement (W-2)

3. Before taking any major actions, such as selling a house, weigh the merits of waiting until age 65, when many special breaks are available to the elderly or retired.
4. Determine the status and duration of ongoing financial commitments such as mortgages and loans.
5. Prepare detailed cash flow projections from estimated year of retirement until age 90, taking inflation into consideration.
6. Practice living for a month under the planned retirement income.
7. Consider different retirement locations. If a location other than the present home is chosen, try living there for a while before making the move.

RIGHT BEFORE RETIREMENT

1. Establish what your retirement income will be, and estimate as closely as possible what your retirement costs of living will be.
2. Have your employer's personnel officer determine exactly what your pension benefits will be, what company or bank will send the pension, and when the first check (or lump-sum distribution) will arrive; what can be done about accumulated vacation time; whether there are any special annuity benefits; and whether supplemental medical or hospital insurance is available.
3. Register with the Social Security Administration at least three months before retirement.
4. Inquire about possible entitlements to partial pensions from past jobs.

RETIREMENT ACTION PLAN

Current Status

Needs Action	Okay or Not Applicable	
☐	☐	1. You must begin to plan for retirement now—it's never too early. Begin by preparing projections of your retirement income and expenses. If you are within ten years of retirement, prepare these projections annually.
☐	☐	2. You cannot rely on pension and Social Security benefits alone to provide for an adequate retirement. Therefore, get into the habit of setting aside some money each year that is earmarked solely for retirement. An IRA (whether or not it is deductible) is an inexpensive and effective means of starting to get into this habit.
☐	☐	3. If you change jobs, roll over any vested pension benefits into an IRA immediately—no matter how small the amount may be and no matter how badly you want to use the money to buy something.
☐	☐	4. If you, like many health-care professionals, are self-employed or practice in a group, set up a retirement plan that is appropriate to your circumstances and needs. You may want to consult with a pension specialist to make sure you adopt the right kind of plan and set it up correctly.
☐	☐	5. If you have any net income from moonlighting (even if you are covered by a pension plan where you work), set up a Simplified Employee Pension (SEP) Plan or a Keogh Plan to contribute tax-deductible money for retirement.

Needs Action	Okay or Not Applicable	
☐	☐	6. One of the best things you can do during your working years to prepare for retirement is to be mortgage free by retirement age. If you are a renter or will still have a large mortgage when you retire, remember that you will need a considerably larger nest egg to cover your housing costs.
☐	☐	7. Review your retirement plan investments periodically. Be sure to consider them in conjunction with your entire investment portfolio—personal investments as well as retirement plan investments.

Comments:_____

_____

_____

_____

_____

_____

Retirement "To Do" List:_____

_____

_____

_____

_____

_____

8

Estate Planning
Checkup

Estate planning is hardly the most exciting topic to discuss. You may think estate planning is only for the very wealthy or the very dead. Actually, every adult, married or single, rich or not-so-rich, needs to pay some attention to estate planning. Most of us don't like to think about estate planning for a couple of reasons. First, since you should invariably involve attorneys in helping you with your estate plans, you're likely to run across some complicated and confusing terminology, such as intestacy (sounds like someone who is missing some organs), codicil (sounds like a fish), QTIP trust (sounds like a trust you put in your ear), and durable power of attorney (sounds like you're authorizing your lawyer to send you bills for the rest of your life). The second reason is that estate planning invariably forces us to think about our own mortality. While they say "only the good die young," and that may assure you a long life, the fact is that no one has yet lived forever.

What is estate planning? It is the process of organizing your financial and personal interests, in accordance with prevailing laws, so that *your* wishes are met with a minimum of inconvenience to your family. Estate planning can also assure that your estate incurs the minimum possible estate-tax burden. This chapter explains, in English, how you can develop a bare-bones estate plan—if that's all you need—and it will also provide some information on more elaborate techniques that may interest you now or some time in the future. Finally, it contains some tips for you if you are approaching your golden years, or for caring for your parents' financial planning concerns if they are. Effective estate planning need not be complicated, and it has several worthwhile objectives, including:

☐ Minimizing the problems and expenses of probate, avoiding potential family conflicts, where possible;

☐ Providing your spouse with as much responsibility and flexibility in estate management as desired, consistent with potential tax savings;

☐ Providing for the conservation of your estate and its effective management, following death of either or both spouses;

☐ Minimizing taxes at time of death as well as income taxes after death;

☐ Avoiding leaving the children too much, too soon;

☐ Providing for adequate liquidity to cover taxes and other expenses at death, without the necessity of forced sale of assets;

☐ Providing for estate management in event of incapacity of either spouse;

☐ Coordinating your personal estate plan with all business arrangements, if applicable;

☐ Organizing all important papers affecting your estate plan in a spot known to all family members, and reviewing them at least annually;

☐ Informing all family members about the overall estate plan.

Physicians, dentists, and other medical professionals often have unique estate planning needs that require special attention. They often accumulate large estates which can benefit from more advanced estate planning techniques. These techniques not only maximize the amount that can be transferred to the next generation, but they also can provide certain benefits during your lifetime.

In spite of the need for estate planning, many health-care professionals are too busy or are not sufficiently informed even to prepare the minimum estate planning documents, or once prepared, to keep them up-to-date. This can cause many problems for the heirs—and, generally, the larger the estate, the greater the problems.

Many health-care professionals are self-employed. The estate planning for self-employed professionals is often more complicated. Among other things, the estate planning must take into consideration the orderly disposition of the professional practice as well as providing sufficient resources to the family during the period following death.

Another matter that may concern health-care professionals is the ability of the family to be adequately prepared to handle a large estate. Again, this potential problem needs to be addressed as part of the estate planning process.

I'm a strong advocate of spending it all before you die—if you have children, you've already done enough for them—but chances are that in spite of your best efforts to follow my recommendation you will end your days with some money left over. Depending upon how much is likely to be left over and your specific wishes as to the disposition of your estate, you at least need to have some basic estate planning documents prepared. Many medical professionals will benefit from some of the optional extras as well.

Example: William and Wilma Willsans were a typical family, two children in grammar school, two cars, one house, one mortgage, and no wills. Will was a laboratory technician, and Wilma was a dental hygienist. Of course, they knew that it was important to have wills, and they intended to get around to it someday. Will died suddenly. Fortunately, he had some life insurance and a few investments that Wilma thought would be sufficient to tide them over for a few years while the family readjusted. She figured that their situation was so typical that she would receive all of the estate, just like they had intended to do in their wills. But such was not the case. The laws of intestate distribution for her state are not unlike many others. Wilma's share of Will's estate is only *one-third*. The other two-thirds goes to the children, and the court must appoint someone to oversee the children's inheritance, because they are minors. So, although Wilma had a serious need for the entire inheritance, she was out of luck. Also, the court will appoint an administrator to carry out the duties of settling Will's estate, which can be much more costly than if an executor had been appointed in a will. Amidst all this chaos, Wilma had better get a will right away, because if she now dies (or if they had died in a common accident), the courts would also appoint guardians for the children, because they had not been designated in a will.

MINIMUM ESTATE PLANNING NEEDS

Estate planning need not be complicated to be effective. A simple estate plan will save legal fees and unnecessary delays and ensure that your estate is distributed in accordance with your wishes. It may also have some positive effects while you are still alive. Unless you want to leave your family in chaos after your demise, take the following minimum steps to provide your loved ones, and yourself, some peace of mind. Single people need to plan their estate as well, because it is highly unlikely that your estate will be distributed in accordance with your wishes upon your demise. For example, many single people want to leave at least a portion of their estate to charity, yet if they die intestate, the charity will never see any of that money. A minimum estate plan usually consists of four documents.

1. VALID AND UP-TO-DATE WILL

Everyone knows the importance of preparing and maintaining a will. Yet the vast majority of adults do not have wills. Your will should specify exactly how your estate is to be divided. It should be drawn up by an experienced attorney. As the above example shows, intestate estates (meaning dying without a will) incur higher than necessary legal fees, unnecessary delays; and a judge, rather than you, will decide how your estate is to be distributed. Changing your will to reflect changes in your personal circumstances (including moving to another state) or changes in state and federal laws is also essential—and often overlooked. Writing a will is simple, but it's not foolproof.

Example: A Simple Will Can Be an Expensive ($235,000) Mistake

Bad idea: The garden-variety will, which in essence says "all to my spouse," could end up costing your children or other heirs a lot of money. Assume a husband has an estate of $1,200,000 (which, by the way, is by no means an unusually large estate for older persons), and he dies leaving all of it to his wife. No federal estate taxes are owed because the transfer qualifies for the unlimited marital deduction. But what if the wife dies right after the husband? She's got at least $1,200,000 to bequeath, but has only the $600,000 tax-free exemption available to reduce estate taxes. Her taxable estate, therefore, is $600,000 (the $1,200,000 gross estate minus the $600,000 exemption). The federal estate tax on this $600,000 is a whopping $235,000, which could have been avoided altogether with some modest estate planning.

Better idea: The husband should limit the wife's taxable estate to the amount covered by her $600,000 exemption, by not willing everything he owns to her. He can do this by allowing her the full use of all of the property to meet her needs, but putting a part of his estate in a trust for her that will not be subject to estate tax at her death.

Of course, the wife might die first, but the estate can be structured to avoid some or all estate taxes no matter who dies first. In the above example, the husband can, during his lifetime, give his wife $600,000 (there are no gift taxes on transfers to a spouse), and she could leave that to him in her will to use if he survives her. Incidentally, these arrangements go under a variety of monikers, including "marital trusts," "A-B trusts," "power of appointment trusts," and (are you ready for this one?) "qualified terminable interest property (QTIP) trusts."

This is but one example of the myriad estate planning opportunities that are available even to persons who somehow missed making the "*Forbes* 400 Richest Americans" list.

Whether you have a will or not (but know you should), the Will Planning and Review Checklist covers important considerations pertaining to the preparation or periodic review of a will.

WILL PLANNING/REVIEW CHECKLIST

This checklist can be used either to plan a new will or review an existing will.

	Current Status			
Yes	No	Unsure	N/A	
☐	☐	☐	☐	1. If there is an existing will, does it reflect the current situation, including birth of heirs and changes in the tax laws, and not contain obsolete sections, including state or residence and executor suitability?
☐	☐	☐	☐	2. Will any specific bequests or legacies be made?
☐	☐	☐	☐	3. Are there any bequests to charity, either outright or in trust, in order to obtain benefit of the charitable deduction?
☐	☐	☐	☐	4. Has the disposition of personal property—furniture, jewelry, and automobiles, for example—been planned?
☐	☐	☐	☐	5. Has provision been made for the disposition of real estate?
☐	☐	☐	☐	6. Does the will provide for the disposition of property if an heir predeceases?
☐	☐	☐	☐	7. Will trusts be established for certain beneficiaries, or will they receive the assets outright?
☐	☐	☐	☐	8. Will certain beneficiaries be provided with periodic payments of income?
☐	☐	☐	☐	9. Does the will take advantage of the unlimited marital deduction to the most effective and practical extent allowed?

Yes	No	Unsure	N/A	
☐	☐	☐	☐	10. Has consideration been given to providing for marital and nonmarital trusts in the will?
☐	☐	☐	☐	11. Is the custody of minors satisfactorily addressed?
☐	☐	☐	☐	12. Has consideration been given to appointing a "financial" guardian for the children in addition to a "personal" guardian?
☐	☐	☐	☐	13. Does the will specify that any minor beneficiary's share of the estate will be held until he reaches maturity?
☐	☐	☐	☐	14. Does the will provide for a guardianship or trust to protect the inheritance of disabled or incompetent beneficiaries?
☐	☐	☐	☐	15. Have provisions been made to dispose of business interests?
☐	☐	☐	☐	16. Have appropriate and capable persons or institutions been appointed to serve as executor, trustee, and/or guardian?
☐	☐	☐	☐	17. Does the will name an alternate or successor executor, trustee, and/or guardian?
☐	☐	☐	☐	18. Should any special powers be given to or taken away from the executor?
☐	☐	☐	☐	19. Has the executor's bond requirement been waived?
☐	☐	☐	☐	20. Are specific powers granted to the executor, as necessary, such as to retain or sell property, to invest trust and estate assets, to allocate receipts and disbursements to income and principal, to make loans and borrow funds, or to settle claims?
☐	☐	☐	☐	21. Is the ownership of the assets complementary to the provisions of the will (that is, some assets may pass outside of the will by contract or by type of ownership)?
☐	☐	☐	☐	22. Does the will state who will receive property if the beneficiary disclaims it? (Disclaimers can be an effective postmortem planning device.)

Yes	No	Unsure	N/A		
☐	☐	☐	☐	23.	Have any special directions for the funeral or memorial been provided?
☐	☐	☐	☐	24.	Have sources been identified from which debts, funeral expenses, and estate administrative costs will be paid?
☐	☐	☐	☐	25.	Will the survivors have enough cash to pay ordinary family living expenses while the estate is in probate?

An experienced lawyer can help you draw up a will to specify exactly how you want your estate divided. Your will does not prevent you from doing whatever you like with your property while you're still alive, and if your circumstances change, you can always write a new one.

2. Durable power of attorney

As if death isn't hard enough to contemplate, the second essential estate planning document will become indispensable in the event you become incapacitated and unable to manage your financial affairs because of an accident, illness, or age. Your right to manage your own affairs may be revoked by a court order, and a guardian will be appointed. It is possible that the court will not appoint the guardian that you would have chosen, and the difficulties in securing court approval of the guardian's actions will create undue red tape and confusion. There are basically two ways to protect personal assets and ensure that they will continue to be managed as you see fit. You can appoint a guardian for yourself by assigning a durable power of attorney, or you can establish a living trust.

Assigning a durable power of attorney ensures that if you ever become unable to manage your own financial and personal affairs, someone that you trust will be able to act on your behalf. A power of attorney may be either special, applying to only certain situations, or general, giving the attorney-in-fact virtually limitless control over the principal (the person who created the arrangement). General powers of attorney should be avoided because they are dangerous, subject to abuse, and usually unnecessary.

A power of attorney may also be either indefinite or for a specific length of time. No matter how it is assigned, it may be cancelled at any time, and it terminates immediately upon the death of the principal. Your state may not recognize durable powers of attorney. If so, you can use a living trust to protect you in the event of incapacity. Since living trusts can accomplish more than a durable power of attorney, you may want to consider a living trust in lieu of a durable power. They are discussed in the Trusts section below.

Also, consider appointing a financial guardian in addition to a personal guardian for your children, in order to separate the responsibility of managing your child's finances from the responsibility of raising your child. This may be particularly desirable if you have a large estate.

3. LIVING WILL

Now that we've taken care of your death and incapacity, we can move on to another dismal topic. You are undoubtedly aware of the medical dilemmas surrounding terminally ill patients and the importance of trying to accommodate the patient's wishes. If you are concerned about these matters personally, you should consider drafting a so-called "living will," informing family members and physicians that under certain circumstances you do not wish to be kept alive by artificial means. You get to define the circumstances. Living wills are legally recognized in most states, and even where they are not, experts suggest that preparing one anyway can be very helpful, if and when the need to make these difficult decisions arises.

4. LETTER OF INSTRUCTIONS

A letter of instructions is not as crucial as other essential estate planning documents, but you will be doing your heirs a big favor by preparing one. A letter of instructions is an informal document (you don't need an attorney to prepare it) that gives your survivors information concerning important financial and personal matters. Although it does not carry the legal weight of a will, the letter of instructions is very important because it clarifies any further requests to be carried out upon death, and provides essential financial information, thus relieving the surviving family members of needless worry and speculation. The

---

It's 10:00 P.M. . . . Do your heirs know where your letter of instructions is?

Letter of Instructions Checklist will help you decide what to include.

Obviously, your survivors will benefit if you prepare a letter of instructions. But you will, too, insofar as a well-prepared letter of instructions is a great way to organize your personal records. Be sure to keep it up-to-date, since the information contained therein is likely to change. Finally, make sure your heirs know where the letter is, before they ever need it. Perhaps you should tape it to your refrigerator door so everyone will know where it is located!

LETTER OF INSTRUCTIONS CHECKLIST

It's really up to you what you want to put in your letter of instructions. Since a letter of instructions is not a legal document like a will, you have a lot more leeway in both the language and content. Your letter is a good place to put personal wishes and final comments, but your heirs will be very grateful if you include some more useful information. The following is a list of suggestions for what to put in your letter of instructions. Even if you're not planning to die in the near future, preparing a letter of instructions is a good way to start getting your records in order. Your heirs will also be very grateful.

☐ *FIRST THINGS TO DO*
- Acquaintances and organizations to be called, including Social Security, the bank, your employer
- Arrangements to be made with funeral home
- Lawyer's name and telephone
- Newspapers to receive obituary information
- Location of insurance policies

☐ *CEMETERY AND FUNERAL*
- Details of your wishes and any arrangements you have made

☐ *FACTS FOR FUNERAL DIRECTOR*
- Vital statistics, including your full name, residence, marital status, spouse's name, date of birth, birthplace, father's and mother's names and birthplaces,

length of residence in state and in United States, military records/history, Social Security number, occupation, and life insurance information

☐ *INFORMATION FOR DEATH CERTIFICATE AND FILING FOR BENEFITS*
- Citizen of, race, marital status, name of next of kin (other than spouse), relationship, address, and birthplace

☐ *EXPECTED DEATH BENEFITS*
- Information about any potential death benefits (including life insurance, profit sharing, pension plan, or accident insurance), life insurance companies, Social Security, the Department of Veterans Affairs, or any other source

☐ *SPECIAL WISHES*
- Anything you want them to know

☐ *PERSONAL EFFECTS*
- A list of who is to receive certain personal effects

☐ *PERSONAL PAPERS*
- Locations of important personal documents, including your will, birth and baptismal certificates, communion and confirmation certificates, diplomas, marriage certificate, military records, naturalization papers, and any other documents (e.g., adoption, divorce)

☐ *SAFE-DEPOSIT BOX**
- Location and number of box and key and an inventory of contents

☐ *POST OFFICE BOX*
- Location and number of box and key (or combination)

☐ *INCOME TAX RETURNS*
- Location of all previous returns
- Location of your estimated tax file
- Tax preparer's name

☐ *LOANS OUTSTANDING*
- Information for loans other than mortgages, including bank name and address, name on loan, account number, monthly payment, location of papers and payment book, collateral, and information on any life insurance on the loan

☐ *DEBTS OWED TO THE ESTATE*
- Debtor, description, terms, balance, location of documents, and comments on loan status/discharge

*State law may require the bank to seal the deceased's box as soon as notified of his death, even if the box is jointly owned.

☐ *SOCIAL SECURITY*
- Full name, SS number, and the location of Social Security card

☐ *LIFE INSURANCE*
- Policy numbers and amounts, location of policy, whose life is insured, insurer's name and address, kind of policy, beneficiaries, issue and maturity date, payment options, and any special facts

☐ *VETERANS*
- If you are a veteran, give information on collecting benefits from local Veterans Affairs office

☐ *OTHER INSURANCE*
- If any other insurance benefits or policies are in force, including accident, homeowner's/renter's, automobile, disability, medical, personal or professional liability, give insurer's name and address, policy number, beneficiary, coverage, location of policy, term, how acquired (if through professional or other group), agent

☐ *INVESTMENTS*
- Stocks: Company, name on certificates, number of shares, certificate numbers, purchase price and date, and location of certificates
- Bonds/notes/bills: Issuer, issued to, face amount, bond number, purchase price and date, maturity date, and location of certificates
- Mutual funds: Company, name on account, number of shares or units, and location of statements and certificates
- Other investments: For each investment, list amount invested, to whom issued, maturity date, issuer, and other applicable data, and location of certificates and other vital papers

☐ *HOUSEHOLD CONTENTS*
- List of contents with name of owners, form of ownership, and location of documents, inventory, and appraisals

☐ *AUTOMOBILES*
- For each car: Year, make, model, color, identification number, title in name(s) of, and location of title and registration

☐ *IMPORTANT WARRANTIES, RECEIPTS*
- Location and description

☐ *DOCTORS' NAMES, ADDRESSES, AND TELEPHONES*
- Including dentist, children's pediatrician, and children's dentist

☐ *CHECKING ACCOUNTS*
- Name of bank, name on account, account number, and location of passbook (or receipt) for all accounts

☐ *CREDIT CARDS*
- For each card: Company (including telephone and address), name on card, number, and location of card

☐ *HOUSE, CONDO, OR CO-OP*
- About the home: in whose name, address, legal description, other descriptions needed, lawyer at closing, and locations of statement of closing, policy of title insurance, deed, and land survey
- About the mortgage: held by, amount of original mortgage, date taken out, amount owed now, method of payment, and location of payment book, if any (or payment statements)
- About life insurance on mortgage: policy number, location of policy, and annual amount
- About property taxes: amount and location of receipts
- About the cost of house: initial buying price, purchase closing fee, other buying costs (real estate agent, legal, taxes), and home improvements
- About improvements: what each consisted of, cost, date, and location of bills
- For renters: lease location and expiration date

☐ *FUNERAL PREFERENCES*
- Specify whether *or not* you would like to have any of the following done: Donate organs, autopsy if requested, simple arrangements, embalming, public viewing, least expensive burial or cremation container, or immediate disposition. Remains should be: donated (details of arrangements made), cremated (and the ashes: scattered, buried at), disposed of as follows (details), or buried (at)
- Specify which of the following services should be performed: memorial (after disposition), funeral (before disposition), or graveside to be held at: church, mortuary, or other
- Specify where memorial gifts should be given or whether or not to omit flowers
- If prearrangements have been made with a mortuary, give details

☐ *SIGNATURE AND DATE*

The four documents described above—a will, durable power of attorney, a living will, and a letter of instructions—are the essential components of a basic estate plan. You may well be able to benefit from other estate planning techniques, including trusts, gifts to relatives, and selecting the appropriate form of property ownership.

OPTIONAL EXTRAS THAT CAN BENEFIT YOU IN THE HERE AND NOW (AS WELL AS THE HEREAFTER)

Many medical professionals have or will accumulate sizable estates. Generally, if your estate is expected to be close to or in excess of $1 million, you may benefit from some of the estate planning techniques that are described below. This may seem like a king's (or a neurosurgeon's) ransom at this point in your life, but if you project your estate into the future, you probably will achieve these lofty levels. How, you might ask, can you figure out the current size of your estate? The following work sheet will allow you to make a quick, albeit rough, estimate of the value of your estate.

QUICK ESTIMATE OF ESTATE VALUE

1. Net worth (from Statement of Personal Assets
   and Liabilities at end of Chapter 1) $.........
2. Life insurance and other death benefits $.........
3. Minus cash value of life insurance listed
   on Statement of Personal Assets and
   Liabilities (to avoid double counting)   (.........)
4. Total life insurance and other death benefits (Line 2 minus Line 3)   ....
      Estimated current value of estate (Line 1 plus Line 4) $.........

TRUSTS

Trusts have a variety of advantages. As I've mentioned before, you don't necessarily have to be a billionaire, or even a millionaire, to take advantage of them. Trusts can increase administrative convenience, shelter you from lawsuits and creditors, allow for a speedier inheritance, and in some cases, reduce

---

Some trusts that are set up for children require that they annually be given a choice either to withdraw money from the trust or waive their power of withdrawal. These are often referred to as "hammerlock" trusts because, if necessary, the parents encourage the child to sign the waiver by applying a hammerlock.

your tax burden at the same time. Most importantly, a trust can be tailored to meet almost all of your objectives. For example, a simple will typically gives your assets to your heirs outright. Many people, particularly those who have accumulated or will accumulate a relatively large estate, are uncomfortable with the prospect of their children receiving all these assets at once, with no strings attached. A trust can be set up that will empower the trustee to distribute trust income to beneficiaries in accordance with their needs. This may be particularly useful if you have a disabled child or if you have children of widely differing economic circumstances.

A trust can be created to shift the burden of management to a trusted third party, to transfer property to minors without the need to appoint a guardian, to safeguard your principal against unwise or extravagant spending during your lifetime, or even as a retirement tool to ensure that you will have a well-managed fund should you become incapable of managing it yourself.

REVOCABLE LIVING TRUSTS

A revocable living trust (sometimes called *inter vivos*), is a useful estate planning tool. A living trust is usually set up to hold your property, naming yourself as the principal beneficiary. Regardless of your age or mental condition, the trustee is legally bound to act in the beneficiary's best interests according to the trust's instructions. A living trust's immediate advantage is that it can minimize or circumvent probate; if all the grantor's assets are held in the trust, there is nothing to transfer through the will. The trust ensures continuous management of the assets, uninterrupted by death. If the grantor at any point is disabled or otherwise unable to make an important decision concerning the assets, the cotrustee can take responsibility. The grantor can appoint a financial adviser as cotrustee if he does not wish to manage all the assets while living. A trust provides more assurance than a will that the grantor's desires will be carried out; a trust document can specify exact conditions about the distribution of assets—such as at what age a child will receive an inheritance—and can allow the trustee the discretion to withhold or distribute extra assets, if prudent or necessary. A living trust is particularly desirable if you live in a state where the probate laws are burdensome.

Some people may be unwilling to establish a living trust, but still want to control the way in which the beneficiaries receive the estate after his or her death. This can be accomplished by creating a trust with instructions contained in your will, known as a "testamentary trust." An example of the use of a testamentary trust was illustrated in the example at the beginning of this section entitled "A Simple Will Can Be An Expensive ($235,000) Mistake." If you set up a revocable living trust or a testamentary trust, you can change or eliminate it during your lifetime.

IRREVOCABLE TRUSTS

Unlike the revocable trust, an *irrevocable* trust requires you permanently to give up the assets you transfer to it. Since the property in trust is no longer yours, it will be transferred on your death to your heirs, without the delays and administrative costs of probate. The best property to put into an irrevocable trust is that which has appreciation potential, because if the property increases in value after you transfer it to the trust, the increase will not be subject to any estate tax. On the other hand, irrevocable trusts incur legal and administrative fees, and most importantly, you lose control of the assets forever. Therefore, these trusts are suitable only if you can easily afford to part with the assets.

GIFTS TO RELATIVES

You can give $10,000 to any person or any number of persons each year without any gift-tax implications. If you are married and funds are coming from jointly held property, or if the spouse consents when the funds are coming from separately held assets of the donor, couples can transfer a total of $20,000 per donee per year without gift-tax consequences.

Consequently, it is possible to reduce the size of your estate significantly, through a program of annual gifts to family members. It is sometimes advisable to make gifts in excess of the $10,000 annual exclusion. When property is owned that is likely to appreciate significantly in value, it may be wise to utilize the $600,000 unified credit for a lifetime gift in order to remove the appreciating asset from the estate before its value increases significantly.

Although your children would love for you to give them a lot of money each year, you must make sure that you have sufficient resources to last you for the rest of your life. How much is sufficient? Generally, if your estate is less than $1,500,000, you should avoid giving any but nominal annual gifts to your children and grandchildren. Why so much? A long-term confinement in a nursing home can reduce the size of a retired person's estate dramatically—even to the point of impoverishing the elderly person or couple.

CHARITABLE GIVING

There is a lot more to charitable giving than simply writing out a check to a favorite charity. In fact, there are a variety of ways to donate property to charity in exchange for a lifetime income for you. In addition, you get a partial income tax deduction—the longer you expect to receive income, the smaller the tax deduction when you donate the cash or property. Finally, these arrangements can result in a deduction in the donor's estate taxes. The most common way for affluent people to garner these benefits is by utilizing one or more types of charitable trusts.

CHARITABLE REMAINDER TRUSTS

A charitable remainder trust is a present gift of a future interest in income-producing property. For example, you could donate securities to a favorite charity in return for an income stream for a specified period of time, such as a set number of years, your lifetime, or the joint lifetimes of you and your spouse. After your death, the property that you originally donated goes to the charity. Donors to a charitable remainder trust can structure the income payments as a set amount or as a fixed percentage of the assets in the trust.

A *pooled income fund* is a particularly convenient charitable remainder arrangement. The assets you contribute to a pooled income fund are comingled with the contributions of others. The donors are paid income from their proportionate shares of the fund, based upon the fund's rate of return. This charitable remainder arrangement is particularly attractive for persons who have a lot of their wealth tied up in one or a few issues of stock, because of the diversification afforded by donating the shares to the much larger pooled-income fund. Whatever assets you intend to contribute, it is important to check out the track record of a fund before making a donation.

Personal financial planning would be a lot easier if we knew when we were going to die.

CHARITABLE LEAD TRUSTS

A charitable lead trust, also known as a front trust or charitable income trust, allows you to contribute the income portion of income-producing property for a certain period of time. Then the assets in the trust revert to your beneficiaries (typically family members). In effect, this is the opposite of a charitable remainder trust. It is especially appropriate for people who have sufficient income, but who want to pass income-producing assets on to future generations. Charitable lead trusts are most useful in gift- and estate tax planning and offer only limited income tax planning opportunities. The best assets to place in these trusts are those with a consistent current yield and significant appreciation potential.

ADDITIONAL TECHNIQUES

Charitable remainder trusts and charitable lead trusts both allow the donor to receive partial income tax deductions and estate tax savings while retaining an interest in the donated property. Other strategies that accomplish these objectives include contributions of partial interests in property (more liberal rules apply to property donated for conservation purposes) or remainder interests in a personal residence or farm, and sales of appreciated property to a charity for less than its current value (so-called "bargain sales"). Many charitable institutions now offer either immediate pay or deferred annuities in exchange for donated property. These charitable gift annuities are often well worth considering. Some people have made good use of the above-mentioned charitable giving arrangements to provide additional income during retirement; but remember, you must be charitably inclined, because better returns can be obtained from other investments.

COMMONLY MADE MISTAKES IN ESTATE PLANNING

Dying without a will or not properly structuring a large estate through the use of trusts are not the only mistakes that can be made in estate planning. This is why it is so essential for you to use the services of a competent estate planning attorney, and don't be surprised if, at some point, you outgrow your family attorney's capability to handle your estate planning matters. Medical professionals who have larger estates need to retain attorneys who work on estate planning matters full time. They are expensive, but the cost of a botched estate will surely be many times greater—although you probably won't be around to witness the effects. The following list describes commonly made estate planning mistakes.

■ While jointly held property may be satisfactory for a relatively small estate, there are a number of potential disadvantages, including a potential double federal estate tax and lack of control over the property once it has passed to the survivor(s). There may be lifetime disadvantages to jointly held property as well, particularly in situations where there is a potential for personal liability arising out of either personal or professional acts.

■ Improperly arranged life insurance can also cause problems in your estate. If your estate is going to be large enough to incur estate taxes, you should consider the use of an *irrevocable life insurance trust*. At a minimum, you need to assure that ownership and beneficiary designations on all of your life insurance policies are appropriate, in view of your personal wishes and from an estate tax planning standpoint.

■ Another problem you may overlook in your estate planning is the need for sufficient liquidity to meet the obligations occasioned by your demise, including probate and administration costs, estate taxes (federal and state), and costs of supporting your family for a period of time after your death. What you need to do is to figure out how much cash and what resources that are readily convertible into cash will be available were you to die today, and compare that with the estimated needs of your family and your estate.

■ Choosing the wrong executor can also create enormous problems, particularly if the chosen individual is inexperienced or may cause friction among family members. So pay particular attention to choosing an executor who can adequately handle the settlement of your estate or who is wise enough to seek professional assistance.

■ If you own property in more than one state, you could create a nightmare for your survivors because it may require probate proceedings in each of the states in which you own property. A properly structured living trust could alleviate this problem. Check with your estate planning attorney.

■ Self-employed doctors and other medical professionals must also assure that funds will be available to ensure an orderly continuation or winding down of the practice.

ADVANCE PLANNING FOR YOUR ADVANCED YEARS (AND CARING FOR YOUR PARENTS IN THEIRS)

Although we often think of ourselves as a nation of materialists who are unwilling to sacrifice our own comfort to take care of our parents, an estimated seven to eight million Americans provide personal care to their parents, so the evidence suggests that Americans do care for their elders. But few of us plan ahead effectively and prepare for the probability that our parents will, at least to some extent, rely on us during their old age, and we, too, will eventually reach an age where we need the assistance of others to carry on our day-to-day activities. In any case, for emotional and financial reasons, anyone with an elderly parent should think about possible action to take if a crisis should happen, so that even if the worst does take place, the consequences will not be needlessly disruptive. Besides, you can plan for your own senior years while you plan for your parents'. You're still too young to worry about such matters? That's the point! For now, we'll start with caring for your parents.

Even an elderly parent who appears to be in good health may be having difficulties that require your help. Unpaid bills, unfilled prescriptions, an overdrawn bank account, or other indications of bouts of forgetfulness are all possible first signs that an elderly person's ability to take care of him- or herself may be lessening. If you've noticed any impairments in your elderly parents, encourage them to be checked thoroughly by a doctor. Although you may be inclined to believe the problem is a natural result of aging, it may well be treatable. Many elderly people resist medical evaluation, often out of fear that they may be sent to a nursing home on the basis of the results, so be sure to assure your parents that they will not be forced to make any changes in their life without their own consent.

While parents are still healthy, it is important that you have a frank discussion with them about plans for and worries about the future. Housing, and the possibility of moving if the present location is inconvenient, is a critical topic. Many retirement homes and other elder-care facilities have long waiting lists. To avoid having an elderly parent placed in an unsatisfactory home because of a sudden illness, you and your parents should discuss alternatives and possibly apply to a home before the need actually arises. Even if your parents are healthy, they should consider any housing decisions in anticipation of possible future health problems.

One of the most important things to plan in advance is how your parents expect to meet any major health-care costs. Do they have sufficient health insurance? Remember that Medicare has many gaps in its coverage. It is difficult but prudent to raise the unpleasant issue of what will happen if your parents become incapable of managing their own affairs. They—as well as you— should have durable powers of attorney or similar documents prepared. Ask your parents how well they have been meeting expenses, keeping in mind that they may not wish to reveal any financial problems. Also, be sure your parents have a file, kept in a location known to you, containing copies of their wills, insurance policies, real estate papers, past tax returns, and other important documents.

The elderly parent's future financial situation also needs to be evaluated. Even an elderly parent who is presently financially secure may eventually run into trouble. A retiree's typically fixed income is always in danger of having its purchasing power eroded by inflation; and, of course, medical care and nursing care can reduce anyone's income and savings drastically. It is important to consider what measures you are willing or able to take to assist your parent financially. Even if you are willing to give some of your own money to your parents, you should discuss with them how they are currently managing their own investments. Many elderly people either invest too conservatively or are susceptible to exploitation by unscrupulous individuals.

Many children live a considerable distance away from their parents, which may make assuring that they are well cared for especially difficult. Most cities have agencies available to meet the basic needs of the elderly, from home health care to companionship and escort services. The National Association of Area Agencies on Aging, 600 Maryland Ave, SW, West Wing, Suite 208, Washington, DC 20024, lists local agencies. You can write NAAAA to request information on agencies in your parents' locale. Services that can be arranged include:

- Emergency medical response systems
- Daily visits by local residents
- Home care (laundry, housecleaning, cooking, small repairs, errands, snow shoveling)
- Legal assistance
- Hot meals (at neighborhood centers or delivered to the home)
- Transportation services
- Day care centers

Further help can be sought through senior citizens' centers, religious organizations, welfare services, nursing homes, local branches of the United Way, and major hospital social services departments or elderly outreach programs. If the elderly person requires substantial health-related assistance, a hospital-based social worker is often the best alternative. Of course, in choosing among these plans, parents should be included in all discussions to the extent possible. By all means, make yourself available to assist your elderly parents with any questions or concerns they may have, and remind them regularly of your willingness to help them at any time.

One final comment pertaining to your parents—or you, if you're elderly. The biggest fear that elderly people have today is that they will be wiped out financially if they have to go into a nursing home. This fear often precipitates drastic financial action. You are probably aware of the efforts many elderly take— often at the urging of their children—to rearrange their assets so they can qualify for Medicaid if they have to enter a nursing home. Parents and children should ask themselves if it is worth having the elderly person enter a Medicaid nursing home in order to pass on some assets to children, or if it is preferable to use these assets, if necessary, to provide a more satisfactory nursing home environment for the parent.

After reading this chapter, you may still be reluctant to take the action necessary to plan your estate. After all, even though your occupation may make you aware of the inevitability of incapacity, terminal illness, and death, you don't want to think about them happening to you or your parents. Nevertheless, I can promise you that you will feel better after having attended to these important matters, and once you have done so, any future changes in your circumstances or plans will be easy to incorporate in your estate planning documents.

ESTATE ACTION PLAN

Needs Action	Okay or Not Applicable	
☐	☐	1. Determine your wishes for the ultimate disposition of your estate.
☐	☐	2. Write an up-to-date will that is consistent with your personal wishes and circumstances.
☐	☐	3. Name an appropriate executor.
☐	☐	4. Prepare and keep up-to-date a letter of instructions.
☐	☐	5. Establish a durable power of attorney or living trust that protects you in the event of incapacity.
☐	☐	6. Designate guardians for your children, and if applicable, disabled adults.
☐	☐	7. Prepare a living will.
☐	☐	8. Prepare an estimate of your taxable estate.
☐	☐	9. Determine if your estate is sufficiently liquid to meet all needs; if not, take action to increase its liquidity.
☐	☐	10. Make sure that the title in which you hold property is appropriate.
☐	☐	11. Any gifts to relatives or charitable contributions should be consistent with your financial condition and overall estate planning.
☐	☐	12. If you own property in more than one state, take appropriate actions to minimize probate problems upon your demise.
☐	☐	13. Consider the use of revocable and irrevocable trusts as part of the estate planning process.

Current Status

Needs Action	Okay or Not Applicable	
☐	☐	14. If you own a practice or other closely held business, make provisions for its disposition in the event of your death.
☐	☐	15. Inform your family and any other beneficiaries of your plans.
☐	☐	16. Consider the possibility that you will incur substantial uninsured health care costs during retirement.
☐	☐	17. If you have elderly parents, inquire as to the status of their personal finances and estate plans.
☐	☐	18. Be sure that the attorney who handles your estate planning is up to the task. If your estate is quite large or complex, you should retain a highly qualified and experienced estate planning attorney.

Comments:_____

_____

_____

_____

_____

_____

Estate Planning "To Do" List:_____

_____

_____

_____

_____

_____

9 Achieving Financial Peace of Mind in the 1990s and Beyond: Ten (Relatively) Simple Things to Do

There are so many important matters to attend to in your personal finances that at times it seems overwhelming. You can't do everything, of course, but there are always some things that you can do to improve your financial well-being. Good personal financial planning doesn't have to be a time consuming, daily process. No one in your profession has much spare time, anyway. Fortunately, there are several basic guidelines that will help you focus on important financial planning and money management matters. I don't promise you financial nirvana, but if you adhere to the following ten financial planning guidelines, you will be able to enjoy some peace of mind, knowing you are well on your way to financial security.

1. *Be happy with what you've got.* People who overextend themselves usually do so in an attempt to maintain a life-style beyond their means. The only way to accumulate wealth is to live *beneath* your means, and the only way to live beneath your means comfortably is to be happy with what you've already got.

2. *Adjust your financial planning to the new realities of the health-care industry.* The economic outlook for the health-care industry in this country ranges from bland to bleak. Many doctors and dentists, in particular, may experience a declining income. Newly minted medical professionals will not enjoy the incomes that their predecessors have enjoyed. You should analyze your career and income prospects realistically, and if necessary, adjust your financial plans to reflect the new reality.

3. *Close all gaps in your insurance coverage.* A single gap

in your insurance coverage could easily wipe out years of savings and investments, or worse. Everyone needs comprehensive and continuous insurance coverage.

4. *Save at least 10 percent of your income (hopefully more).* It is inexcusable not to save at least 10 percent of your *gross* income (not net), no matter what your circumstances. If you say you can't do it, you haven't looked hard enough at how you spend your money. Unless you inherit it or marry it, you will never accumulate enough money to achieve retirement security without saving regularly.

5. *Maintain a balanced investment portfolio that is appropriate to your own financial situation.* Most people invest in extremes, either taking too much risk or too little risk. The best portfolio structure is one that includes stock investments, interest-earning investments, and perhaps, real estate investments. Your chosen asset allocation should be considered a long-term allocation, one that is not altered materially in response to current market conditions, or worse, the opinions of some "experts."

6. *Develop a reasonable investment strategy and stick with it.* Fill your balanced investment portfolio with sensible (some might say dull) investments that you wouldn't mind holding for the rest of your life. Don't overlook the many advantages offered by mutual funds. Above all, be consistent in carrying out your investment strategy.

7. *Don't let income tax saving considerations outweigh more important financial planning matters.* Some people haven't yet learned that the tax reform of the 1980s has reduced the importance of tax deductions considerably. Current rules require a new and better way of thinking. Rather than asking, "Is this going to save me taxes?" you should ask, "Is this a worthwhile cost or investment?"

8. *Recognize that it will cost a fortune to retire comfortably, and begin preparing now.* Much of what you do in your year-to-year financial planning is directly or indirectly geared toward assuring you a comfortable retirement. Yet many people still fall short. No matter how young or old you are, don't delay projecting your retirement needs and planning to meet them. Take advantage of the many tax-deferred, retirement-earmarked savings plans available.

9. *Prepare and keep up-to-date necessary estate planning documents (unless you dislike your heirs).* If you are one of the many who don't yet have a will, durable power of attorney, and a living will, by all means ask an attorney to prepare them. Believe it or not, you will feel better for having done so. Higher income or

net worth medical professionals may benefit from more sophisticated estate planning techniques.

10. *Take control of your personal finances.* Don't rely too much on others (including myself) to tell you what is good for your own situation. You know best. Medical professionals are very busy people, but you still need to devote at least some time to managing your money and your advisers.

Good financial planning begins with good common sense. Financial security may still be a long way off, but as you begin to take control of your financial future, you'll find that many rewards accompany the sacrifices along the way. Don't get discouraged, and always remember that *you* are your own best financial planner. Good luck!

FINANCIAL PLANNING "THINGS TO DO TOMORROW" LIST

Before you put this book away, please write down three things that you need to do *now* to help improve your personal finances. The three things don't need to be the most crucial; instead they should be matters that you can accomplish with relative ease, like arranging with your bank to have some money automatically and regularly withdrawn from your checking account and placed in a savings or investment account. After you have accomplished these three tasks, you'll be encouraged to do more, and you'll be well on your way to a successful financial life.

1. _____

2. _____

3. _____

Take Control Over Your Financial Future

Now that you're ready to take control of your financial future, you're ready for **SMART PLANNER**. **SMART PLANNER** is an innovative approach to individual financial analysis that gives you a personalized report on your unique financial needs. Developed by Jonathan Pond, **SMART PLANNER** provides useful recommendations to help you in all the areas covered in this book, including:

- Saving
- Investing
- Real estate
- Insurance
- Retirement planning
- Record keeping
- Income taxes
- Budgeting
- Education planning
- Estate planning

Your personalized **SMART PLANNER** report will show you how to:

- Save more in order to assure financial security
- Make the right kind of investments to meet your financial goals
- Avoid making financially crippling mistakes
- Take immediate action to assure a comfortable retirement
- Assure you will be cared for if you are disabled
- Avoid having a judge decide who should inherit your estate

SMART PLANNER is:

- *Unbiased*   **SMART PLANNER** is not affiliated with any financial institution. Its analysis and recommendations are completely objective.
- *Customized*   Your report addresses your specific financial status and needs. Persons of all ages and income levels benefit from **SMART PLANNER** since each report is unique.
- *Easy to Understand*   You are assured of receiving up-to-date information in everyday language.
- *Confidential*   Information from your questionnaire and report is held in the strictest confidence.
- *Realistic*   **SMART PLANNER** provides down-to-earth recommendations, not "get rich quick" schemes.
- *Guaranteed*   If you are not completely satisfied with your **SMART PLANNER** report, your money will be refunded promptly.

IT'S EASY TO RECEIVE YOUR PERSONAL *SMART PLANNER* REPORT.

1. After ordering **SMART PLANNER**, you will receive a confidential financial planning questionnaire. The questionnaire is easy to fill out. You will not have to spend hours digging up obscure financial information and filling out confusing financial forms. In fact, most people complete the questionnaire in less than 30 minutes.
2. Send the completed questionnaire back to the data center. Your responses are then processed and your individualized report is prepared.
3. Your personalized **SMART PLANNER** report is sent to you by first-class mail within two weeks. The report presents a comprehensive and objective review of your financial situation in all areas of personal finance. Age, family status, and income information provided in the questionnaire allow **SMART PLANNER** to tailor the report to your unique financial needs.

Every bit of valuable information in your 20 to 25 page report pertains to you and you alone. Plus, it comes with a list of *recommendations* in order of importance so you will know exactly which items are most essential to your financial security and *work sheets* so that you can start to take action to improve your financial status.

ORDER *SMART PLANNER* TODAY

When you're ready to order **SMART PLANNER,** send a check for $39.95 to

SMART PLANNER, 9 Galen Street, Watertown, MA 02172

or call 1 (800) 448-8112 with your MasterCard or VISA ready. Massachusetts residents add 5% sales tax for a total of $41.95.